Taping, Wrapping, and Bracing for Athletic Trainers

Functional Methods for Application and Fabrication

T0198131

Taping, Wrapping, and Bracing for Athletic Trainers

Functional Methods for Application and Fabrication

Editor

Andy Grubbs, MEd, ATC
Director of Athletic Training
The Hughston Foundation
Columbus, Georgia

Associate Editors

Ryan P. Barbier, MS, LAT, ATC, NREMR
Certified Athletic Trainer, South Larouche High School
Cut Off, Louisiana

Jonathan P. Born, MS, LAT, ATC
Certified Athletic Trainer, Johnson High School
Atlanta Rehabilitation and Performance Center
Gainesville, Georgia

D. Alexander King, LAT, ATC
Certified Athletic Trainer, Etowah High School
Children's Healthcare of Atlanta
Woodstock, Georgia

Megan A. Purk, MS, LAT, ATC
Certified Athletic Trainer
Bowling Green, Missouri

Wm. Chad Witzel, MS, LAT, ATC, ITAT
Certified Athletic Trainer, Meade County High School
Hardin Memorial Hospital
Elizabethtown, Kentucky

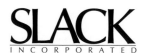

SLACK
INCORPORATED

www.Healio.com/books

ISBN: 978-1-61711-983-5

The procedures and practices described in this publication should be implemented in a manner consistent with the professional standards set for the circumstances that apply in each specific situation. Every effort has been made to confirm the accuracy of the information presented and to correctly relate generally accepted practices. The authors, editors, and publisher cannot accept responsibility for errors or exclusions or for the outcome of the material presented herein. There is no expressed or implied warranty of this book or information imparted by it. Care has been taken to ensure that drug selection and dosages are in accordance with currently accepted/recommended practice. Off-label uses of drugs may be discussed. Due to continuing research, changes in government policy and regulations, and various effects of drug reactions and interactions, it is recommended that the reader carefully review all materials and literature provided for each drug, especially those that are new or not frequently used. Some drugs or devices in this publication have clearance for use in a restricted research setting by the Food and Drug and Administration or FDA. Each professional should determine the FDA status of any drug or device prior to use in their practice.

Any review or mention of specific companies or products is not intended as an endorsement by the author or publisher.

SLACK Incorporated uses a review process to evaluate submitted material. Prior to publication, educators or clinicians provide important feedback on the content that we publish. We welcome feedback on this work.

Published by: SLACK Incorporated
                             6900 Grove Road
                             Thorofare, NJ 08086 USA
                             Telephone: 856-848-1000
                             Fax: 856-848-6091
                             www.Healio.com/books

Contact SLACK Incorporated for more information about other books in this field or about the availability of our books from distributors outside the United States.

Library of Congress Cataloging-in-Publication Data

Names: Grubbs, Andy, editor.
Title: Taping, wrapping, and bracing for athletic trainers : functional
    methods for application and fabrication / editor, Andy Grubbs ; associate
    editors, Ryan P. Barbier, Jonathan P. Born, D. Alexander King, Megan A.
    Purk, Wm. Chad Witzel.
Description: Thorofare, NJ : SLACK Incorporated, [2017] | Includes
    bibliographical references and index.
Identifiers: LCCN 2016039324 (print) | LCCN 2016039831 (ebook) | ISBN
    9781617119835 (pbk. : alk. paper) | ISBN 9781630914141 (epub) | ISBN
    9781630914158 (web)
Subjects: | MESH: Athletic Injuries--rehabilitation | Athletic Tape |
    Compression Bandages | Braces | Sports Medicine--methods
Classification: LCC RD97 (print) | LCC RD97 (ebook) | NLM QT 261 | DDC
    617.1/027--dc23
LC record available at https://lccn.loc.gov/2016039324

Printed in the United States of America.

Last digit is print number: 10 9 8 7 6 5 4 3 2 1

DEDICATION

This is dedicated to all the individuals who have attended the Hughston Foundation Athletic Training Fellowship Program and to all our families and friends involved in the application, development, and finalization of this book.

CONTENTS

Acknowledgments

Many individuals deserve recognition and thanks for their assistance in developing *Taping, Wrapping, and Bracing for Athletic Trainers: Functional Methods for Application and Fabrication*. For their time, efforts, and careful review of this manuscript, we would like to thank the following Hughston Foundation staff members:

- Belinda Klein, MA, Executive Director and Director of Medical Imagery
- Tiffany Davis, MS, Medical Illustrator
- Robbie Ross, Director of Medical Television
- Christine Maisto, PhD, CMT, Medical Writing and Editing
- Dennise Brogdon, Medical Writer

ABOUT THE EDITOR

Andy Grubbs, MEd, ATC joined the Hughston Foundation as Director of Athletic Training in June 2010. His primary responsibility is oversight of the 18 graduate assistant athletic trainers who provide medical care to the local area high schools and professional sports teams. He received his Bachelor of Science degree in athletic training from Valdosta State University in 2001 and a master's degree in education from Auburn University in 2003. Prior to coming to Hughston, Mr. Grubbs worked at South Effingham High School in Rincon, Georgia, and The University of West Alabama in Livingston, Alabama.

ABOUT THE ASSOCIATE EDITORS

Ryan P. Barbier, MS, LAT, ATC, NREMR's interest and eventual career in athletic training began in high school with the involvement and encouragement of Bart Folse, the school's head athletic trainer. Mr. Barbier attended Nicholls State University in Thibodaux, Louisiana, where he obtained his Bachelor of Science degree in athletic training. He was then accepted into the 2-year athletic training fellowship program at the Hughston Foundation in Columbus, Georgia. While there he obtained his Master of Science degree in physical education from the University of North Georgia. Currently, Mr. Barbier is teaching sports medicine and medical terminology and is an emergency medical responder in Central Louisiana high schools.

Jonathan P. Born, MS, LAT, ATC is the head athletic trainer of Johnson High School in Gainesville, Georgia. Mr. Born received his Bachelor of Science degree in athletic training from the University of North Georgia in Dahlonega, Georgia. Mr. Born then took his skills to the Hughston Foundation in Columbus, Georgia, as an athletic training fellow where he worked with Chattahoochee Valley Community College in Phenix City, Alabama. There he assisted with their softball, men's and women's basketball, and 2-time ACCC Champion baseball team. While in Columbus, Mr. Born received his master's degree in physical education from the University of North Georgia.

D. Alexander King, LAT, ATC is the head athletic trainer at Etowah High School in Woodstock, Georgia, as an employee of Children's Healthcare of Atlanta. Mr. King's beginnings in athletic training came at Union College (Kentucky) under the direction of then-program director Clay Butler, the college's director of sports medicine and head athletic trainer. Working with the '09 World Series Baseball team at Union and gaining first-hand experience in a field that genuinely helped others while being immersed in a very competitive sporting environment, there was no turning back for Mr. King in his career. After earning his Bachelor of Science degree in athletic training, Mr. King began the athletic training fellowship at the Hughston Foundation in Columbus, Georgia, where he has begun his master's degree.

Megan A. Purk, MS, LAT, ATC started her athletic training career at Truman State University in Kirksville, Missouri. She graduated from Truman with a Bachelor of Science degree in athletic training. Following her undergraduate career, Ms. Purk continued her education with the Hughston Foundation in Columbus, Georgia. With the Hughston Foundation she completed a 2-year athletic training fellowship where she worked with Auburn University's club and recreational sports. While she was with the Hughston Foundation, she also received her Master of Science degree in physical education and health from the University of North Georgia. Ms. Purk currently works for Gilmer High School in North Georgia as the health science and sports medicine teacher, as well as the head athletic trainer.

Wm. Chad Witzel, MS, LAT, ATC, ITAT developed his interest in athletic training under the guidance and mentoring of his high school athletic trainer, Terry DiCapio. Mr. Witzel attended Eastern Kentucky University in Richmond, Kentucky, where he obtained his Bachelor of Science degree in athletic training. Following his undergraduate studies, Mr. Witzel completed a 2-year athletic training fellowship with the Hughston Foundation in Columbus, Georgia. While a fellow, he had the opportunity to work at Auburn University, where he covered club and recreation athletics. Mr. Witzel also obtained his Master of Science degree in physical education and health from the University of North Georgia as a Hughston fellow. Currently, Mr. Witzel works for Hardin Memorial Hospital as a high school outreach certified athletic trainer in Central Kentucky.

About the Contributing Authors

Aubrey Carr, LAT, ATC developed an interest in becoming an athletic trainer after she sustained an injury in gymnastics that required rehabilitation. Ms. Carr received a Bachelor of Science degree in athletic training from Florida State University where she found an appreciation for the mentorships she received from athletic trainer Ms. Eunice Hernandez. Ms. Carr is currently a fellow in the Hughston Foundation Athletic Training Fellowship Program and works as the head athletic trainer at a high school in Columbus, Georgia. She is currently working toward her Master of Science degree in health and physical education and hopes to earn a doctorate degree and teach in an athletic training education program in the future.

Amanda Guethlein, LAT, ATC obtained her Bachelor of Science degree in athletic training from Eastern Kentucky University in Richmond, Kentucky. She is currently obtaining her Master of Science degree in physical education through the University of North Georgia. Ms. Guethlein is a certified athletic trainer in the Hughston Foundation Athletic Training Fellowship Program in Columbus, Georgia. She is currently doing research and assisting with coverage on outside events. After completion of her master's degree, Amanda intends on finding a position in the high school setting or continuing on to physician assistant school.

Adam Norman, LAT, ATC obtained his Bachelor of Science degree in athletic training from Arkansas State University in Jonesboro, Arkansas. Currently obtaining his Master of Science degree in physical education through the University of North Georgia, Mr. Norman is working as a certified athletic trainer for the Columbus Cottonmouths as part of the Hughston Foundation Athletic Training Fellowship Program in Columbus, Georgia. After completion of his master's degree, Mr. Norman intends on finding a position in the collegiate setting.

Mary-Catherine Senn, LAT, ATC is currently working as a graduate assistant athletic training fellow for the Hughston Foundation Clinic in Columbus, Georgia. Upon completion of her Bachelor of Science degree in athletic training, and after earning the Clinical Achievement Award from her CAATE-accredited program, she found Hughston's program to give her the full opportunity to enhance her passion in working as a full-time athletic trainer, along with expanding her skills and understanding of the profession. While Ms. Senn has long-term goals to pursue physician assistant schooling upon completion of her Master of Science degree in physical education, she continues to keep her options open in doing what she absolutely loves, and she looks forward to every opportunity to learn and grow in pursuit of her goals.

PREFACE

Since the inception of the Hughston Foundation Athletic Training Fellowship Program in 1998, several certified athletic trainers have attended from different educational programs and locations, and with different methods of taping and bracing. Each participant in the Hughston Foundation Athletic Training Fellowship Program is to complete a 2-year assistantship, with completion of a Master of Science degree in physical education, in which he or she is exposed to a variety of sporting events requiring different taping and bracing procedures. In 2010, the Hughston Foundation Athletic Training Fellowship Program became the official sports medicine provider for the Muscogee County School District, which allows the fellows to be assigned local schools to provide medical coverage. Throughout the years of the Hughston Foundation Athletic Training Fellowship Program, fellows have demonstrated numerous taping, wrapping, and bracing techniques. *Taping, Wrapping, and Bracing for Athletic Trainers: Functional Methods for Application and Fabrication* provides a unified collection of these techniques.

INTRODUCTION

For many years, sports medicine and health care practitioners have used taping and bracing for both the prevention and rehabilitation of injuries; consequently, specific protocols and techniques have evolved to ensure that the results are functional. To understand the proper taping protocols and techniques and to be able to identify and apply these to athletes and those participating in physical activities, sports practitioners such as athletic trainers, coaches, and allied health care practitioners need both comprehensive knowledge and practical skills. These include training in anatomy and physiology and injury prevention. The National Athletic Trainers' Association has identified a total of 8 different content areas that reflect clinical athletic training practice. In order to become competent athletic trainers, students must master the skills and clinical protocols essential to each content area.

Before discussing the different bracing and taping techniques, it is important to become familiar with the different types of materials available for use. When it comes to athletic tape, there are many choices based on size, color, brand, material, and type of adhesive. Common taping materials include elastic adhesive tape, elastic self-adherent tape, and heavy duty adhesive tape, such as Leukotape (BSN medical Inc), Kinesio tape (Kinesio Holding Corporation), and Cover-Roll (BSN medical Inc), not to mention other types and brands. While this book offers material recommendations for each bracing and taping technique, it is important to understand that some taping techniques can be performed with a number of different types of taping materials.

In the field of athletic training, the most commonly used tape is white athletic tape. This is an adhesive, porous tape that comes in sizes ranging from 0.5 to 3 inches. White athletic tape is also universal and can be easily modified.

Elastic adhesive tape is typically a durable, cloth-like tape. It is most often used in conjunction with white athletic tape to provide a more rigid tape job that lasts longer. Because of its elastic make-up, elastic adhesive tape will expand, and this can help to reduce inflammation because the compression it provides on the injured area prevents significant amounts of swelling. Typically, elastic adhesive tape comes in sizes that range from 1 to 4 inches.

Self-adherent elastic tape is another popular elastic bandage commonly used for wound care and compression. Like white athletic tape, self-adherent elastic tape is porous, and it ranges in size from 1 to 6 inches.

Leukotape is a durable, adhesive tape often used to stabilize joints or reduce range of motion. Leukotape is frequently used as an alternative to or in conjunction with white athletic tape. The benefit of this tape is that it does not tend to loosen up when the person becomes active. As with elastic adhesive tape, this characteristic allows for a more rigid tape job that lasts longer.

Kinesio tape is a newly developed therapeutic tape that has become very popular, especially among volleyball players. The operative principle behind Kinesio tape is to facilitate the body's natural healing system and to provide support and stability to the joints and muscles without restricting range of motion. Some practitioners use Kinesio tape for muscle re-education, pain reduction, and to promote circulation and healing. Lack of knowledge, experience, and research regarding Kinesio tape, as well as its uniqueness, have prompted us to exclude it from this textbook.

Cover-Roll is a thick, porous, elastic tape known for its ability to be modified. Cover-Roll is also hypoallergenic, which makes it a great tool to use for athletes and patients who are sensitive to other kinds of tapes and adhesives. While this tape can be used for a multitude of purposes, it is most often used for first aid, friction reduction, or as a foundation for other tapes.

FUNDAMENTALS OF ALL TAPE JOBS

- Consider what motion you are trying to prevent.
- Consider the materials needed to complete the tape job.
- Don't force the tape to go in a certain direction. Think about where the tape needs to go and angle it accordingly.
- The tape and prewrap should be smooth and relatively wrinkle free.
- Make sure the tape job is comfortable for the athlete.
- Make sure the tape job is functional.
- Always check capillary refill after the tape job is complete.

1

Foot and Ankle

INTRODUCTION AND ANATOMY

The ankle is a commonly injured body part among athletes. The ankle constitutes the foundational support for the body and functions as both a shock absorber and propulsion mechanism. The foot and ankle have 3 main structural components: the forefoot, the midfoot, and the hindfoot.[1] The forefoot contains 5 metatarsals and 14 phalanges and extends up to the tarsometatarsal joint (also called the Lisfranc joint). The metatarsals are numbered, starting medially at the great toe or hallux, which is numbered 1, and continuing laterally to the small toe, which is designated 5. The 5 bones of the midfoot are relatively immobile with respect to one another, but they do provide a mechanical link between the forefoot and hindfoot. The midfoot contains the navicular, the cuboid, and the 3 cuneiforms and extends from the tarsometatarsal joint distally to the transverse tarsal joint proximally.[2] The hindfoot contains the calcaneus and the talus. The calcaneus is the largest tarsal bone and forms the heel of the foot; it also helps support the weight of the body and provides an attachment for muscles to move the foot.[2,3] The superior aspect articulates with the talus via 3 articular surfaces—the anterior, middle, and posterior facets.[2] The irregularly shaped talus is also the most superior of the tarsal bones. It is situated superior to the calcaneus over a bony projection called the sustentaculum tali. Because the talus fits into the space formed by the ankle bones or malleoli, lateral movement is restricted by the stabilizing ligaments

Grubbs A, ed.
*Taping, Wrapping, and Bracing for Athletic Trainers:
Functional Methods for Application and Fabrication* (pp 1-62).
© 2017 SLACK Incorporated.

of the ankle. Because the upper-most articular surface of the talus is nar-rower anteriorly than posteriorly, dorsiflexion is limited.[2] The average range of motion is 10 degrees in dorsiflexion and 23 degrees in plantar flexion.[4]

The superior tibiofibular joint is a diarthrotic joint; this means that it allows some gliding movements. By contrast, the inferior tibiofibular joint is a fibrous articulation[5] between the lateral malleolus and the distal end of the tibia. The superior portion of the talus forms a hinge that allows the foot to both dorsiflex and plantar flex. This joint is held together by the anterior tibiofibular ligament that helps prevent excessive separation of the tibia and fibula. The interosseous ligament, which lies superior to the anterior tibiofibular ligament, also assists in preventing excessive separation of the tibia and fibula and can be damaged. This is known as a *high ankle sprain*. The ankle joint, referred to as the *talocrural joint*, is a synovial joint located between the talus, the medial malleolus of the tibia, and the lateral mal-leolus of the fibula. The smooth dome-shaped proximal surface of the talus, the talar dome, is the surface on which the tibia and fibula articulate. On the medial side of the joint, the major ligamentous complex consists of the deltoid or medial collateral ligament of the foot. The deltoid ligament is fan-shaped and resists eversion of the foot and ankle. On the lateral aspect of the joint lies the anterior talofibular, calcaneofibular, and posterior talofibular ligaments. The anterior talofibular ligament prevents excessive inversion while the posterior talofibular ligament resists dorsiflexion, adduction, medial rotation, and medial translation of the ankle. The calcaneofibular ligament provides support to prevent inversion of the ankle.

Many sport activities involve some running, jumping, and changing directions. The foot is in direct contact with the ground, and the forces cre-ated by these athletic movements place a great deal of stress on its structures. Consequently, the foot is associated with a high rate of injury.[5-8]

The foot consists of 26 bones—14 phalanges, 5 metatarsals, and 7 tar-sals. Additionally, there are 2 sesamoid bones beneath the first metatarsal.[5] The toes are designed to give a wider base for balance and for propel-ling the body forward. The first toe or hallux has 2 phalanges and the other toes each have 3. Two sesamoid bones are located beneath the first metatarsophalangeal joint. They help reduce pressure during weightbearing, increase the mechanical advantage of the flexor tendons of the great toe, and act as a pulley for tendons.[5]

The intrinsic foot muscles originate on the foot and directly influence the motion of both the foot and toes. By contrast, the extrinsic foot muscles originate on the lower leg and/or the distal femur. The extrinsic muscles also help produce motion at the foot and ankle.[9]

The foot's intrinsic muscles originate and insert from the foot and are grouped into 4 layers based on their depth in the foot.[2,9] The first and most superficial layer includes the abductor hallucis, flexor digitorum brevis, abductor digiti minimi, and plantar aponeurosis. All of these muscles originate from the calcaneus and attach onto the phalanges.[2,9] The second or middle layer contains the quadratus plantae, the tendons of the flexor hallucis longus, and the lumbricals; the flexor digitorum longus tendons also pass through the middle layer. The third or deep layer of the intrinsic muscles consists of the flexor hallucis brevis, the adductor hallucis, and the flexor digiti minimi brevis. The final layer, the interosseous layer, contains the plantar and dorsal interossei. These muscles assist in adducting the lateral 3 toes and abducting the middle 3 toes.[2,9]

The extrinsic muscles that help to move the foot arise from the compartments of the lower leg. These muscles include the flexor hallucis longus, which aids in plantar flexing, adducting, and supinating the foot and ankle. The flexor digitorum longus also plantar flexes the ankle while supinating the foot. The extensor hallucis longus and extensor digitorum longus help in ankle dorsiflexion and extension of the 4 phalanges. The extensor digitorum longus also contributes slightly to ankle pronation.[2,9]

The 3 arches of the foot function as shock absorbers to buffer and dissipate ground reaction forces as well as to increase foot flexibility. The medial arch is formed by the articulation of the calcaneus, talus, navicular, first cuneiform, and first metatarsal. The medial arch helps to allow a greater range of motion than the other 2 arches. It also gains muscular support from the calcaneonavicular or spring ligament, the long and short plantar ligaments, the deltoid ligaments, and the foot's plantar fascia. The lateral longitudinal arch is lower and more rigid than the medial arch. It is composed of the calcaneus, the cuboid, and the fifth metatarsal and injury to this area is very rare. The transverse metatarsal arch is formed by the lengths of the metatarsals and tarsals and is shaped by the concave features of the metatarsals. It originates at the metatarsal heads and continues to the calcaneus. Structurally, the transverse arch is supported by the medial and longitudinal arches as well as by the peroneus longus muscle.[9]

COMMON INJURIES

Toe

Hyperextension (Turf Toe)

Turf toe is a hyperextension of the flexor ligament of the great toe[1,5]

Mechanism of Injury

- Often associated with the use of flexible footwear or artificial turf[1]
- Flexible footwear is often worn on turf, resulting in more dorsiflexion of the toe[5]
- Commonly injured and exacerbated during push-off phase of running, sprinting, or jumping[5]
- Commonly seen in track, football, volleyball, and soccer

Common Signs and Symptoms

- Tenderness at the great toe joint[5]
- Pain with extension of the great toe[5]
- Mild to moderate inflammation[5]

Hyperflexion (Soccer Toe)

Soccer toe is a hyperflexion of the extensor ligament of the great toe

Mechanism of Injury

- Frequently injured when the great toe is folded underneath the foot during activity
- Commonly seen after striking a soccer ball, the toe drags on the ground, resulting in hyperflexion
- Commonly seen in soccer and kickers in football

Common Signs and Symptoms

- Tenderness at the great toe joint
- Pain with flexion of the great toe
- Mild to moderate inflammation

Bunion

- A deviation at the first metatarsophalangeal joint, often caused by inflammation of a bursa or hallux valgus, causing medial protrusion of the metatarsophalangeal joint and lateral shift of the great toe[9]
- Callus formation, thickened bursa, and exostosis are the 3 phases of bunion development[1,5]

Mechanism of Injury

- Often caused by wearing shoes with improper toe box size, resulting in repetitive constriction of the toes[9]
- Can also be a genetic anomaly
- Commonly seen in women who frequently wear high heels or soccer players who wear smaller cleats
- Can also be caused by hallux valgus[1,5,9]

Common Signs and Symptoms

- Protrusion of the metatarsophalangeal joint of the great toe medially[9]
- Lateral shift of the great toe[9]
- Tenderness at the metatarsophalangeal joint[5]
- Mild to moderate inflammation[5]

Bunionette

A deviation of the fifth metatarsophalangeal joint, causing lateral protrusion of the metatarsophalangeal joint and medial shift of the fifth phalanx[9]

Mechanism of Injury

- Often caused by wearing shoes with improper toe box size, resulting in repetitive constriction of the toes
- Can also be a genetic anomaly
- Commonly seen in women who frequently wear high heels or soccer players who wear smaller cleats

Common Signs and Symptoms

- Protrusion of the fifth metatarsophalangeal joint laterally[1,9]
- Medial shift of the fifth phalanx[5,9]
- Tenderness at the metatarsophalangeal joint[5]
- Mild to moderate inflammation[5]

Morton's Neuroma

A neuroma between the third and fourth metatarsal

Mechanism of Injury

- Irritation of the nerve bundle between the third and fourth metatarsal
- Commonly seen in track and cross country runners and dancers

Common Signs and Symptoms

- Pain on the plantar aspect of the foot
- Mild inflammation in the forefoot
- Athlete presents with pain while weightbearing on the ball of the foot

Foot

Plantar Fasciitis

Irritation of the plantar fascia or the tendon sheath[5,9]

Mechanism of Injury

- Single traumatic episode[9]
- Repetitive stress[9]
- Biomechanical deficits[9]
- Possible heel spur[5,9]
- Nerve entrapment[9]
- Achilles tendon tightness[9]
- Changes in activity intensity and duration[9]
- Weight gain[9]
- Improper footwear[5]

Common Signs and Symptoms

- Point tender in the posterior aspect of arch[5]
- More prominent pain in the morning or after nonweightbearing[5]
- Increased pain when using stairs[9]
- Walking barefoot[9]
- Tightness over the Achilles tendon and gastrocnemius[9]

Falling Arch Syndrome (Flatfoot)

Genetic abnormality or traumatic onset to a tendon, resulting in lowering of the medial longitudinal arch

Mechanism of Injury

- Genetic
- Traumatic episode
- Biomechanical deficits
- Improper footwear

Common Signs and Symptoms

- Pain in the medial longitudinal arch
- Increased Q-angle
- Possible referred pain into the knees or hips
- Possible great toe involvement
- Increased pronation resulting in tight peroneals

Lisfranc Injury (Ligament Sprain or Tear, Fracture, Dislocation)

Injury to any of the tarsal ligaments

Mechanism of Injury

- Injury is often caused by low-energy forces (sprain) or axial loading while the toes are extended causing high-energy force (fracture/dislocation)

Common Signs and Symptoms

- Sprain
- Palpable pain over midfoot
- Potential mild inflammation
- Fracture/dislocation
- Severe palpable pain
- Visible deformity
- Rapid onset of inflammation

Ankle

Inversion (Lateral) Ankle Sprain

Injury to the anterior talofibular ligament, calcaneofibular ligament, or posterior talofibular ligament caused by a sudden traumatic force[9] or by sudden inward rolling of the foot and ankle resulting in ligamentous injury[9]

Mechanism of Injury

- Commonly caused by inversion, plantar flexion, and internal rotation resulting in ligamentous sprain or rupture[5]

Common Signs and Symptoms

- Rapid inflammation[5,9]
- Discoloration[5,9]
- Decreased range of motion[5,9]
- Decreased muscular strength[9]
- Palpable tenderness over the talar dome, sinus tarsi, and lateral aspect of the ankle[5,9]
- Gait abnormality[5,9]

Eversion (Medial) Ankle Sprain

Injury to the deltoid ligament caused by a sudden traumatic force[5,9]

Mechanism of Injury

- Sudden traumatic force causing the excessive external rotation of the ankle[9]

Common Signs and Symptoms

- Rapid localized inflammation[9]
- Discoloration[9]
- Decreased range of motion[9]
- Palpable tenderness over deltoid ligament or medial joint line of the ankle[5,9]
- Gait abnormality[9]

Syndesmotic (High) Ankle Sprain

Injury to the tendon sheath and/or interosseous ligament

Mechanism of Injury

- Sudden traumatic force causing the excessive external rotation and dorsiflexion of the ankle and the fibula to separate from the tibia[9]

Common Signs and Symptoms

- Inflammation[9]
- Decreased range of motion[9]
- Palpable tenderness over talar dome and the interosseous ligament[5,9]
- Gait abnormality[9]

Achilles Injuries (Strain/Tendinitis)

Injury to the Achilles tendon[5]

Mechanism of Injury

- Tightness of the triceps surae due to overuse[5,9]
- Single traumatic force, excessive dorsiflexion[5,9]
- Improper footwear[9]
- Biomechanical deficits

Common Signs and Symptoms

- Possible visible edema[9]
- Involved tendon may appear thicker than on the opposite leg[9]
- Pain,[5,9] stiffness,[5] or burning along the length of the tendon
- Crepitus (popping or crunchy feeling)[5,9]
- Tightness along the gastrocnemius and soleus[5,9]
- Gait abnormalities[9]

TAPE JOBS

Toes

Great Toe

Turf Toe

Materials Needed

- Adhesive spray (apply prior to taping)
- 1-inch white athletic tape
- 1.5-inch white athletic tape

Step 1

Apply adhesive spray to targeted taping area (Figure 1-1-1).

Figure 1-1-1.

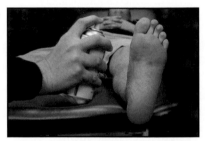

Step 2

With the 1.5-inch white athletic tape, place an anchor strip around the midfoot proximal to the metatarsal head (Figure 1-1-2).

Figure 1-1-2.

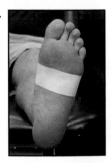

Step 3

With the 1-inch white athletic tape, place an anchor strip around the great toe (Figure 1-1-3).

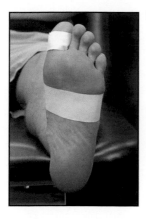

Figure 1-1-3.

Step 4

Make a fan out of the 1-inch white athletic tape (Figure 1-1-4).

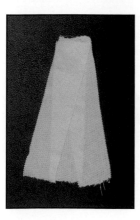

Figure 1-1-4.

Step 5

Anchor the fan to the great toe using 1-inch white athletic tape (Figure 1-1-5).

Figure 1-1-5.

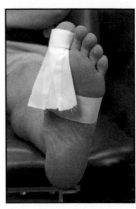

Step 6

Pulling proximally toward the midfoot, anchor the fan, using 1.5-inch white athletic tape (Figure 1-1-6).

Figure 1-1-6.

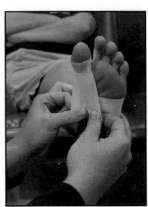

Step 7

Close tape job with C strips (Figure 1-1-7).

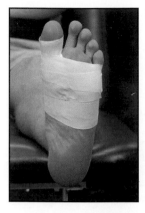

Figure 1-1-7.

Step 8

Check for capillary refill (Figure 1-1-8).

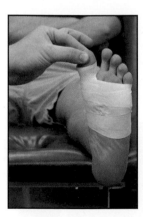

Figure 1-1-8.

Please refer to the Turf Toe tape job (Video) for further review and variation preference in performing this taping technique.

Toe Spica

Materials Needed

- Adhesive spray (apply prior to taping)
- Prewrap (optional)
- 1-inch white stretch tape
- 1.5-inch white athletic tape

Step 1

Apply adhesive spray to targeted taping area (Figure 1-2-1).

Figure 1-2-1.

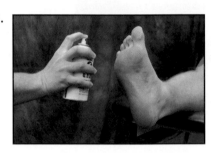

Step 2

Place a C strip along the plantar surface of the foot at the base of the metatarsals and then a separate C strip along the dorsal aspect of the foot to serve as an anchor (Figure 1-2-2).

Figure 1-2-2.

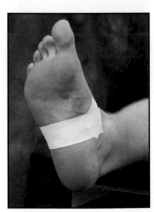

Step 3

Using 1-inch stretch tape, pull out a strip that is long enough to reach from the plantar midfoot, around the toe, to the dorsal midfoot. Place the middle of the tape strip around the medial aspect of the great toe (Figure 1-2-3).

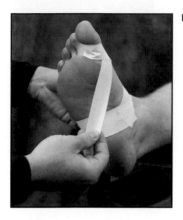

Figure 1-2-3.

Step 4

With equal tension on the tape, having wrapped the strips around the toe, cross the strips, attaching one tail strip to the plantar aspect of the midfoot and the other around the dorsal midfoot, across the plantar midfoot, finishing on the dorsal aspect (Figure 1-2-4).

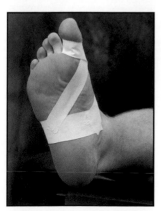

Figure 1-2-4.

Step 5

Repeat Step 3 until the great toe joint is adequately stabilized and functional (Figure 1-2-5).

Figure 1-2-5.

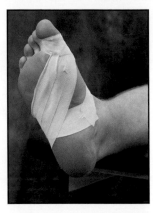

Step 6

Place C strips over the midfoot anchor to close the tape job (Figure 1-2-6).

Figure 1-2-6.

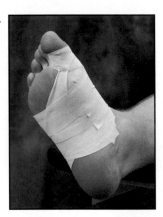

Step 7

Check for capillary refill (Figure 1-2-7).

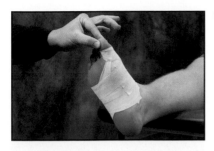

Figure 1-2-7.

Please refer to the Toe Spica tape job (Video) for further review and variation preference in performing this taping technique.

Turf Toe Strap

Materials Needed

- Adhesive spray (apply prior to taping)
- Moleskin straps (premade or custom)
- 1-inch stretch tape
- 3-inch stretch tape

Step 1

Apply adhesive spray to targeted taping area (Figure 1-3-1).

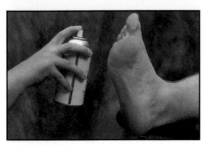

Figure 1-3-1.

Step 2

Attach the distal portion of the moleskin strap around the great toe (Figure 1-3-2).

Figure 1-3-2.

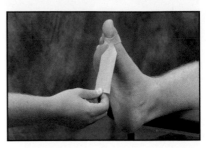

Step 3

Apply tension and pull the strap toward the midfoot, attaching the moleskin (Figure 1-3-3).

Figure 1-3-3.

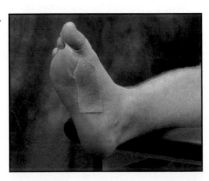

Step 4

Using 1-inch stretch tape, anchor the moleskin to the great toe (Figure 1-3-4).

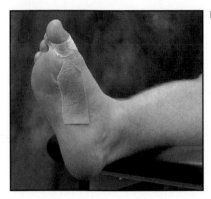

Figure 1-3-4.

Step 5

Then wrap 3-inch stretch tape around the foot, covering the strap and closing the tape job (Figure 1-3-5).

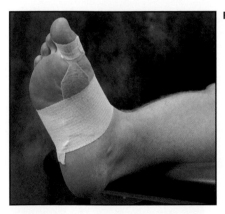

Figure 1-3-5.

Step 6

Check for capillary refill (Figure 1-3-6).

Figure 1-3-6.

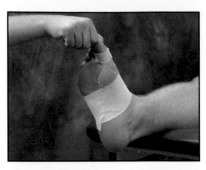

Please refer to the Turf Toe Strap tape job (Video) for further review and variation preference in performing this taping technique.

Foot

Arch

X Arch

Materials Needed

- Adhesive spray (apply prior to taping)
- 1-inch white athletic tape
- 1.5-inch white athletic tape

Step 1

Apply adhesive spray to targeted taping area (Figure 1-4-1).

Figure 1-4-1.

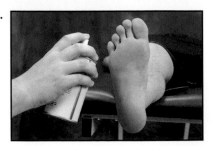

Step 2

Using 1.5-inch tape, place a C strip along the plantar surface of the foot at the metatarsal heads and a separate C strip along the dorsal aspect of the foot at the metatarsal heads to serve as an anchor (Figure 1-4-2).

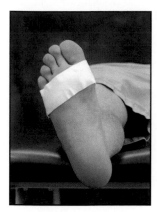

Figure 1-4-2.

Step 3

With 1-inch white athletic tape, start at the plantar aspect of the first metatarsal head, cross the arch of the foot, loop around the calcaneus, and finish by crossing back over the arch and attaching to the plantar aspect of the fifth metatarsal head (Figure 1-4-3).

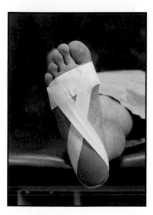

Figure 1-4-3.

Step 4

Then begin at the base of the fourth metatarsal, cross the arch of the foot, loop around the calcaneus, and finish by crossing back over the arch and attaching to the first metatarsal head (Figure 1-4-4).

Figure 1-4-4.

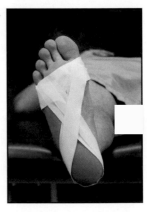

Step 5

Finally, begin at the base of the third metatarsal, cross the arch of the foot, loop around the calcaneus, and finish by crossing back over the arch and attaching to the third metatarsal head (Figure 1-4-5).

Figure 1-4-5.

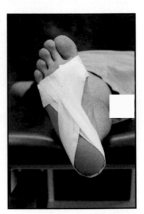

Step 6

Repeat Steps 3 through 5, until the entire plantar surface and medial arch are covered (Figure 1-4-6).

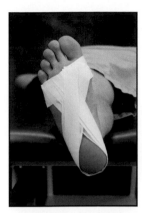

Figure 1-4-6.

Step 7

Apply C strips starting at the metatarsal heads covering to the calcaneus to cover the plantar surface (Figure 1-4-7).

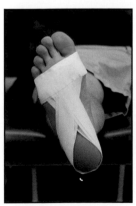

Figure 1-4-7.

Step 8

Lastly, on the dorsal surface of the foot, apply C strips to anchor the tape job, beginning at the metatarsal heads, and closing off the plantar C strips (Figure 1-4-8).

Figure 1-4-8.

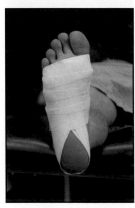

Step 9

Check for capillary refill (Figure 1-4-9).

Figure 1-4-9.

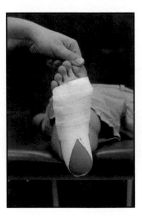

Please refer to the X Arch tape job (Video) for further review and variation preference in performing this taping technique.

Teardrop Arch

Materials Needed

- Adhesive spray (apply prior to taping)
- 1-inch white athletic tape
- 1.5-inch white athletic tape

Step 1

Apply adhesive spray to targeted taping area (Figure 1-5-1).

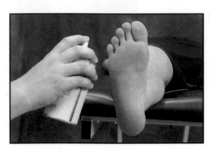

Figure 1-5-1.

Step 2

Place a C strip, with each end split in half to better conform to the foot, along the plantar surface of the foot at the metatarsal heads. Then place a separate C strip along the dorsal aspect of the foot at the metatarsal heads to serve as an anchor (Figure 1-5-2).

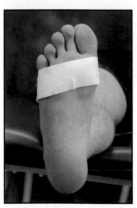

Figure 1-5-2.

Step 3

With 1-inch white athletic tape, start at the first metatarsal head, proceed down the medial plantar surface, loop around the calcaneus, cross over the medial arch, and finish at the starting point of the first metatarsal head (Figure 1-5-3).

Figure 1-5-3.

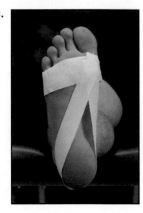

Step 4

Begin at the head of the fifth metatarsal, proceed down the lateral plantar surface, loop around the calcaneus, cross over the medial arch, and finish at the starting point of the fifth metatarsal head (Figure 1-5-4).

Figure 1-5-4.

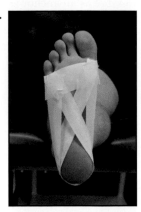

Step 5

Repeat Steps 3 and 4 overlapping by half the tape width until the entire plantar surface and medial arch is covered (Figure 1-5-5).

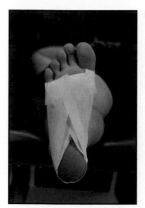

Figure 1-5-5.

Step 6

Start at the metatarsal head and apply C strips with 1.5-inch white athletic tape over the medial arch, covering the plantar surface completely. Apply tension medially (Figure 1-5-6).

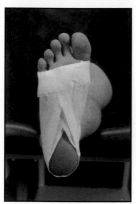

Figure 1-5-6.

Cover the dorsal aspect of the foot with C strips to close out the tape job (Figure 1-5-7).

Figure 1-5-7.

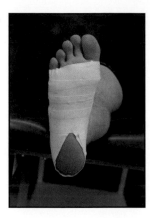

Check for capillary refill (Figure 1-5-8).

Figure 1-5-8.

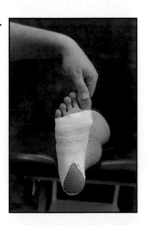

Please refer to the Teardrop Arch tape job (Video) for further review and variation preference in performing this taping technique.

Plantar Fasciitis Strap

Materials Needed

- Adhesive spray (apply prior to taping)
- Moleskin (premade or custom)
- 1.5-inch stretch tape

Step 1

Cut the moleskin into T-type shape (Figure 1-6-1).

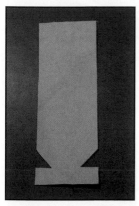

Figure 1-6-1.

Step 2

Apply adhesive spray to targeted taping area (Figure 1-6-2).

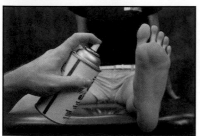

Figure 1-6-2.

Step 3

Beginning on the posterior aspect of the lower leg, attach the proximal end of the strap to the Achilles tendon (Figure 1-6-3).

Figure 1-6-3.

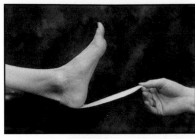

Step 4

Apply distal tension and attach the moleskin down the midfoot to the metatarsal heads (Figure 1-6-4).

Figure 1-6-4.

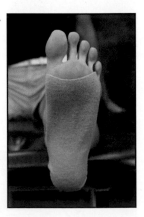

Step 5

Using the 1.5-inch stretch tape, cover the foot and heel (Figure 1-6-5).

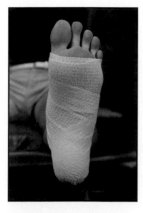

Figure 1-6-5.

Step 6

Check for capillary refill (Figure 1-6-6).

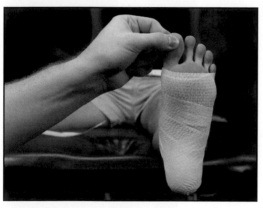

Figure 1-6-6.

Please refer to the Plantar Fasciitis Strap tape job (Video) for further review and variation preference in performing this taping technique.

Ankle

Ankle Tape/Closed Basketweave

Materials Needed

- Adhesive spray (apply prior to taping)
- Heel and lace pads (optional)
- Prewrap (optional)
- 1.5-inch white athletic tape

Step 1

Apply adhesive spray to targeted taping area (Figure 1-7-1).

Figure 1-7-1.

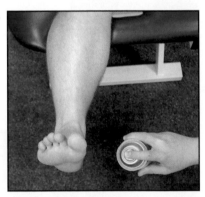

Step 2

Place heel and lace pads as pictured on the distal Achilles and dorsal aspect in the shoelace area (Figure 1-7-2).

Figure 1-7-2.

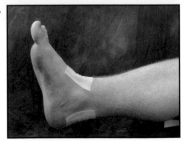

Step 3

Cover with prewrap from inferior gastrocnemius of the lower leg to the midfoot (Figure 1-7-3).

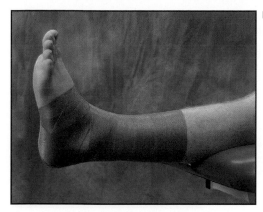

Figure 1-7-3.

Step 4

Place 2 to 3 separate anchor strips inferior to the gastrocnemius, overlapping by half the tape width (Figure 1-7-4).

Note: Angle the tape so that it lies flat against the ankle.

Place another anchor strip at the base of the fifth metatarsal (optional).

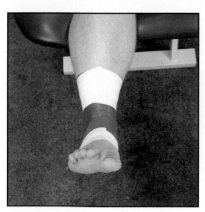

Figure 1-7-4.

Step 5

Start at the medial aspect of the lower leg at the anchor, and place the first stirrup. With lateral pull, pass over the medial malleolus, under the calcaneus, and back to the lateral aspect of the anchor (Figure 1-7-5).

Figure 1-7-5.

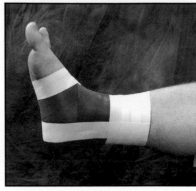

Step 6

Place the first horseshoe around the posterior inferior aspect of the malleolus (Figure 1-7-6).

Figure 1-7-6.

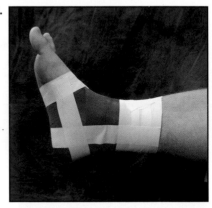

Step 7

Place a second stirrup. Start half the tape's width anteriorly, pulling laterally and slightly anteriorly, pass under the calcaneus, and back to the lateral aspect of the anchor, posterior to the first stirrup. Then place a second horseshoe over the medial malleolus, overlapping the first horseshoe by half the tape's width (Figure 1-7-7).

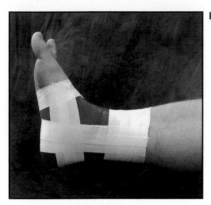

Figure 1-7-7.

Step 8

Place a third and final stirrup, overlapping half the tape's width anteriorly to the first stirrup. Pull laterally and slightly anteriorly, passing under the calcaneus, and back to the lateral aspect of the anchor, anteriorly to the first stirrup. Then place a third and final horseshoe around the posterior superior aspect of the malleolus, overlapping half the tape's width with the previous horseshoe (Figure 1-7-8).

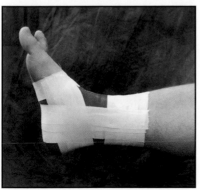

Figure 1-7-8.

Step 9

For the first lateral heel lock, begin at the mortise of the ankle and angle laterally and inferiorly, crossing the lateral malleolus, around the lateral aspect of the calcaneus, and returning posteriorly to the starting point (Figure 1-7-9).

Figure 1-7-9.

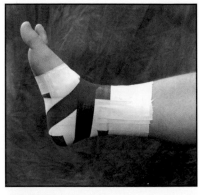

Step 10

For the first medial heel lock, begin at the mortise of the ankle and angle medially and inferiorly, crossing the medial malleolus, around the lateral aspect of the calcaneus, and returning posteriorly to the starting point (Figure 1-7-10).

Figure 1-7-10.

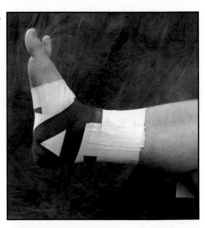

Step 11

For the second medial and lateral heel locks, repeat Steps 9 and 10 (Figure 1-7-11).

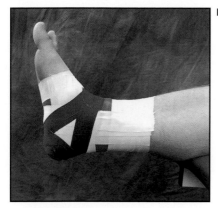

Figure 1-7-11.

Step 12

Starting your figure 8 at the dorsal aspect of the foot, move laterally around the plantar aspect, superolaterally across the ankle mortise, around the posterior ankle, and back to the ankle mortise (Figure 1-7-12).

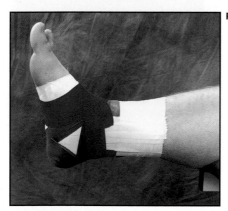

Figure 1-7-12.

Step 13

Repeat Step 12 to complete a second figure 8 (optional; Figure 1-7-13).
Note: More figure 8's can be added to increase stability.

Figure 1-7-13.

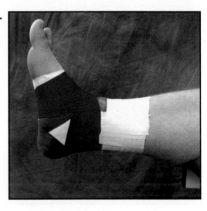

Step 14

Close the tape job using C strips (Figure 1-7-14).

Figure 1-7-14.

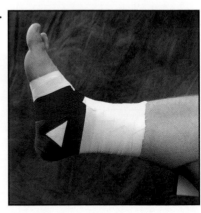

Step 15

Check for capillary refill (Figure 1-7-15).

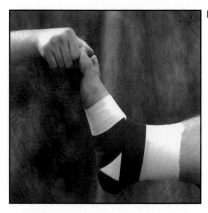

Figure 1-7-15.

Please refer to the Ankle Tape/Closed Basketweave tape job (Video) for further review and variation preference in performing this taping technique.

Spartan

Materials Needed

- Adhesive spray (apply prior to taping)
- Heel and lace pads
- Prewrap (optional)
- 1.5-inch white athletic tape
- 3-inch elastic tape

Step 1

Apply adhesive spray to targeted taping area (Figure 1-8-1).

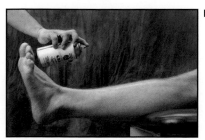

Figure 1-8-1.

Step 2

Apply heel and lace pads to the foot and cover the ankle with pre-wrap from the distal aspect of the gastrocnemius to the arch of the foot (Figure 1-8-2).

Figure 1-8-2.

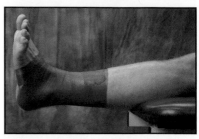

Step 3

Place 2 to 5 separate, slightly angled anchor strips inferior to the gastrocnemius, overlapping by half the tape width (Figure 1-8-3).

Figure 1-8-3.

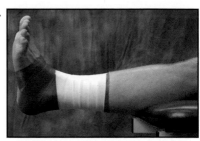

Step 4

Beginning medially, apply 3-inch Elastikon (Johnson & Johnson), pulling medially to laterally under the plantar aspect of the midfoot. Split the lateral piece of Elastikon to create a V, wrapping the posterior strip posteriorly and the anterior strip anteriorly, having the V just inferior to the lateral malleolus (Figures 1-8-4A and B).

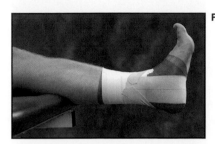

Figure 1-8-4A.

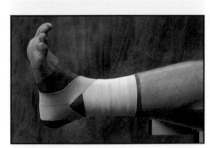

Figure 1-8-4B.

Step 5

Repeat Step 4 on the other side, starting the Elastikon on the lateral aspect of the ankle and placing the V inferior to the medial malleolus (Figures 1-8-5A and B).

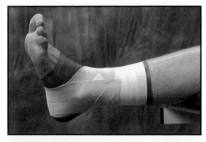

Figure 1-8-5A.

Figure 1-8-5B.

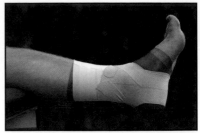

Step 6

Using 1.5-inch stretch tape or 1.5-inch white tape, for the first medial heel lock, begin at the mortise of the ankle and angle medially and inferiorly, crossing the medial malleolus, around the lateral aspect of the calcaneus, and returning posteriorly to the starting point (Figure 1-8-6).

Figure 1-8-6.

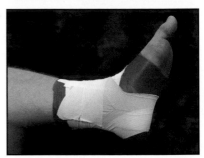

Step 7

For the first lateral heel lock, begin at the mortise of the ankle and angle laterally and inferiorly crossing the lateral malleolus, around the lateral aspect of the calcaneus, and returning posteriorly to the starting point (Figure 1-8-7).

Figure 1-8-7.

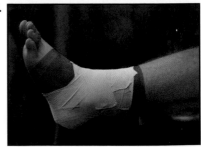

Step 8

For the second medial and lateral heel locks, repeat Steps 6 and 7 (Figure 1-8-8).

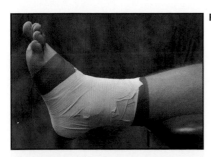

Figure 1-8-8.

Step 9

For the first figure 8, start proximally to the lateral malleolus and move posteriorly around the lower leg, across the anterior mortise, inferolaterally across the base of the fifth metatarsal and midfoot, returning across the anterior mortise to the starting point (Figure 1-8-9).

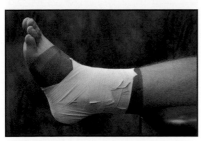

Figure 1-8-9.

Step 10

Repeat Step 9 to complete the second and final figure 8 (Figure 1-8-10).

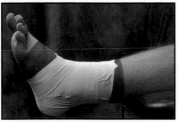

Figure 1-8-10.

Step 11

Close up the tape job. Starting at the level of the malleolus, place closing strips to seal, overlapping each by half the tape's width, until reaching the starting anchor (Figure 1-8-11).

Figure 1-8-11.

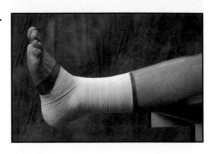

Step 12

Check for capillary refill (Figure 1-8-12).

Figure 1-8-12.

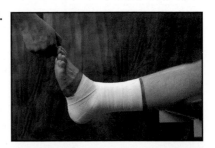

Please refer to the Spartan Ankle Tape tape job (Video) for further review and variation preference in performing this taping technique.

Achilles

Materials Needed

- Adhesive spray (apply prior to taping)
- Prewrap (optional)
- 1.5-inch white tape
- 2- or 3-inch Elastikon tape

Note: Position the athlete either prone or supine, depending on your taping preference.

Step 1

Apply adhesive spray to targeted taping area (Figure 1-9-1).

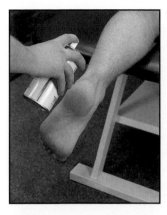

Figure 1-9-1.

Step 2

Starting superior to the base of the gastrocnemius, apply a strip of pre-wrap around the lower one-third of the gastrocnemius and another around the midfoot. Apply 2 to 3 anchor strips over the proximal and distal attachment sites (Figure 1-9-2).

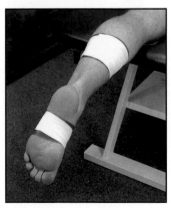

Figure 1-9-2.

Step 3

Premeasure the Elastikon before cutting. Allow about 1 inch extra on both ends to be split and wrapped around (Figure 1-9-3).

Figure 1-9-3.

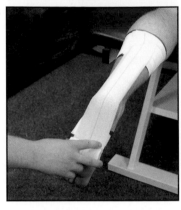

Step 4

Split the proximal end, creating a Y shape, and wrap it around, securing it to the proximal anchor (Figure 1-9-4).

Figure 1-9-4.

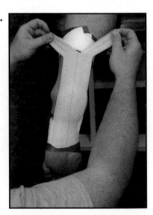

Step 5

With the ankle plantar flexed between 15 and 30 degrees, split and secure the Elastikon around the distal anchor. Apply tension prior to securing to the proximal anchor (Figure 1-9-5).

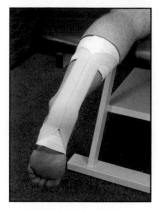

Figure 1-9-5.

Step 6

Repeat Steps 3 through 5 twice more, or until desired support is achieved, overlapping by half the tape's width medially and laterally (Figure 1-9-6).

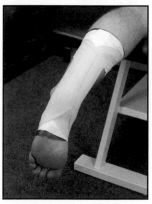

Figure 1-9-6.

Step 7

Place another anchor around the base of the fifth metatarsal and inferiorly to the gastrocnemius (Figure 1-9-7).

Figure 1-9-7.

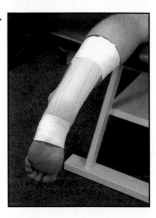

Step 8

Cover with stretch tape to close the tape job (Figure 1-9-8).

Figure 1-9-8.

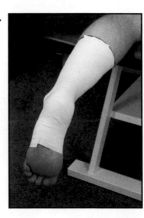

Step 9

Check for capillary refill (Figure 1-9-9).

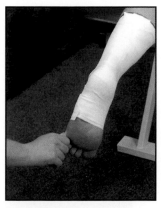

Figure 1-9-9.

Please refer to the Achilles tape job (Video) for further review and variation preference in performing this taping technique.

Braces

Ankle

Air Cast

Materials Needed

- Air cast
- Pump

Step 1

Choose the correct size air cast based on foot size and the manufacturer's sizing chart (Figure 1-10-1).

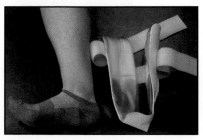

Figure 1-10-1.

Step 2

Loosen the straps and adjust side stirrups to be even with the medial and lateral malleoli (Figure 1-10-2).

Figure 1-10-2.

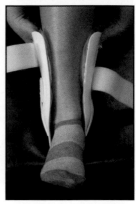

Step 3

Next, tighten the straps around the lower leg until the air cast makes a snug fit (Figure 1-10-3).

Figure 1-10-3.

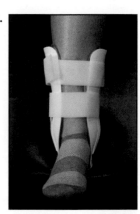

Step 4

Place the foot into the shoe and lace it up. If necessary, adjust the air cast straps to make more snug and/or add air to ensure a snug fit (Figure 1-10-4).

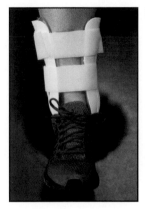

Figure 1-10-4.

Lace-Up

Materials Needed

- Ankle brace

Step 1

Choose the correct size lace-up ankle brace based on foot size and the manufacturer's sizing chart (Figure 1-11-1).

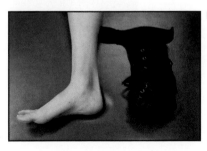

Figure 1-11-1.

Step 2

Loosen laces/straps and place the heel in the calcaneal space (Figure 1-11-2).

Figure 1-11-2.

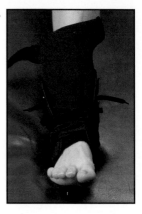

Step 3

Starting at the distal end of the foot, begin to tighten the laces working proximally (Figure 1-11-3).

Figure 1-11-3.

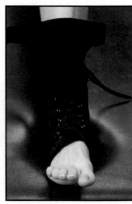

Step 4

If the brace comes with a top strap, tuck the loose ends of the laces under to prevent from loosening and tighten Velcro (Figure 1-11-4).

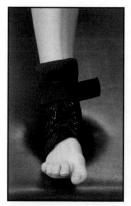

Figure 1-11-4.

Step 5

Once the laces and strap are snugly tied, place the foot into the shoe and adjust to ensure a snug fit (Figure 1-11-5).

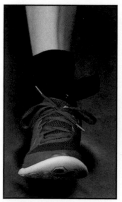

Figure 1-11-5.

Ankle Stabilizing Orthosis ([ASO] Lace-Up Strap Brace)

Materials Needed

- ASO brace

Step 1

Choose the correct size ASO ankle brace based on foot size and the manufacturer's sizing chart (Figure 1-12-1).

Figure 1-12-1.

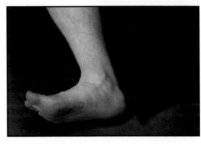

Step 2

Loosen the laces/straps and place the heel in the calcaneal space (Figure 1-12-2).

Figure 1-12-2.

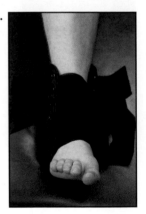

Step 3

Starting at the distal end of the foot, begin to tighten the laces working proximally (Figure 1-12-3).

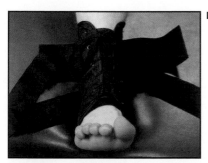

Figure 1-12-3.

Step 4

Once the laces are snugly tied, take the figure 8 straps across the mortise of the foot, under the midfoot, and back across the mortise of the foot and attach to the appropriate medial or lateral Velcro attachment site (Figure 1-12-4).

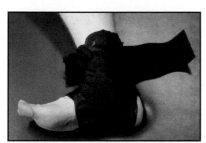

Figure 1-12-4.

Once the figure 8 straps are secure, wrap the closing elastic cuff around the top of the figure 8 straps to secure them in place. The logo should be facing forward (Figure 1-12-5).

Figure 1-12-5.

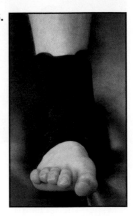

Boot

Materials Needed

- Properly fitted boot

Step 1

Choose the correct boot size based on foot length and the manufacturer's sizing chart, ensuring that the heel is in the proper calcaneal space (Figure 1-13-1).

Figure 1-13-1.

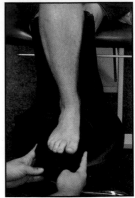

Step 2

Close the Velcro foot covers securely (Figure 1-13-2).

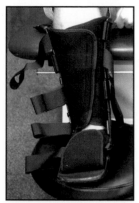

Figure 1-13-2.

Step 3

Begin tightening the straps from the distal to proximal portions of the lower leg (Figure 1-13-3).

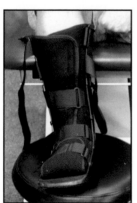

Figure 1-13-3.

Step 4

Begin by tightening the straps distally and working proximally. Tighten the straps until a snug, supportive fit is achieved (Figure 1-13-4).

Figure 1-13-4.

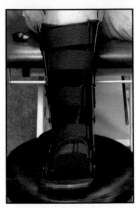

Step 5

Utilize the air pump to ensure a proper and snug fit (Figure 1-13-5).

Figure 1-13-5.

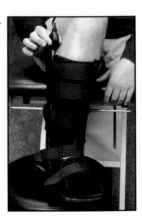

Wraps

Compression Wraps

Ankle Compression Wrap With Horseshoe

Materials Needed

- Compression wrap or stretch tape
- Felt or foam (premade or custom)

Step 1

Beginning on the distal aspect of the foot, apply compression wrap, moving proximally, until reaching the distal aspect of the ankle (Figure 1-14-1).

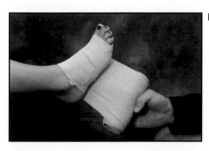

Figure 1-14-1.

Step 2

Place the premade or custom horseshoe over the medial or lateral malleolus (Figure 1-14-2).

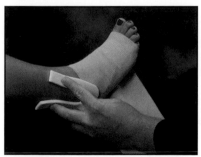

Figure 1-14-2.

Step 3

Secure the horseshoe as you continue to wrap proximally, finishing just above it (Figure 1-14-3).

Figure 1-14-3.

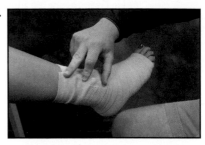

Step 4

Using either the Velcro end of the compression wrap or metal fasteners, secure the proximal end of the compression wrap (Figure 1-14-4).

Figure 1-14-4.

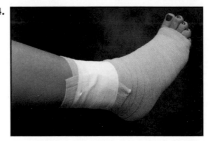

Step 5

Check for capillary refill (Figure 1-14-5).

Disclaimer: The patient should be placed on crutches at this point because functional use of the foot will be limited and warrants limiting weightbearing.

Figure 1-14-5.

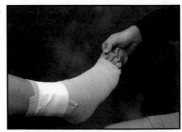

Please refer to the Ankle Compression Wrap tape job (Video) for further review and variation preference in performing this taping technique.

Donut

Materials Needed

- Compression wrap or stretch tape
- Felt or foam (premade or custom)

Step 1

Place the premade or custom donut over the intended area (Figure 1-15-1).

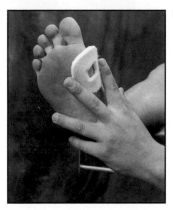

Figure 1-15-1.

Step 2

Beginning on the distal aspect of the foot, use stretch tape to encircle the foot, securing the donut as you continue to wrap proximally (Figure 1-15-2).

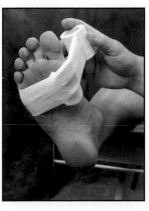

Figure 1-15-2.

Step 3

Check for capillary refill (Figure 1-15-3).

Disclaimer: If elected, compression wrap can be substituted for elastic or self-adhesive tape to secure the donut.

Figure 1-15-3.

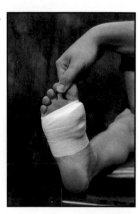

REFERENCES

1. Magee DJ. *Orthopedic Physical Assessment*. 6th ed. New York, NY: Elsevier Health Sciences; 2013.
2. Thordarson D. *Foot and Ankle*. Philadelphia, PA: Lippincott Williams & Wilkins; 2004.
3. Shier D, Butler J. *Hole's Essentials of Human Anatomy and Physiology*. 9th ed. Boston, MA: McGraw-Hill; 2006.
4. Valmassy R. *Clinical Biomechanics of the Lower Extremities*. St. Louis, MO: Mosby; 1996.
5. Prentice WE. *Arnheim's Principles of Athletic Training: A Competency-Based Approach*. 14th ed. New York, NY: McGraw-Hill; 2010.
6. Bruckner P. Foot pain. In: Bruckner P, ed. *Clinical Sports Medicine*. Sydney, Australia: McGraw-Hill; 2002.
7. Jaivin JS. Foot injuries and arthroscopy in sport. *Sports Med*. 2000;29(1):65-72.
8. Sherman KP. The foot in sport. *Br J Sports Med*. 1999;33(1):6-13.
9. Starkey C, Brown SD. *Examination of Orthopedic and Athletic Injuries*. 4th ed. Philadelphia, PA: FA Davis Co; 2015.

Please see videos on the accompanying website at
www.healio.com/books/tapingAT

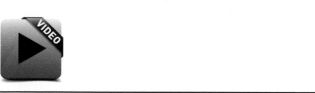

Lower Leg and Knee

INTRODUCTION AND ANATOMY

The lower leg is a major anatomical part of the skeletal system and lies between the knee and the ankle. It contains 2 major long bones, the tibia and the fibula, which are both strong skeletal structures. The tibia is the shinbone, and the fibula is the significantly smaller rear calf bone. The main muscle in this area of the leg is the gastrocnemius muscle, which gives the calf its bulging appearance. The lower leg constitutes a major portion of a person's overall body mass. Its primary functions are standing, walking, running, jumping, and other similar motor activities, even the weightbearing ones. The lower leg is divided into 4 compartments that contain its various muscles. The anterior compartment holds the tibialis anterior, the extensor digitorum longus, the extensor hallucis longus, and the peroneus tertius muscles. These muscles dorsiflex the foot and toes. The tibialis anterior also assists in turning the foot inward. The lateral compartment lies along the outside of the lower leg. It contains the peroneus longus and peroneus brevis muscles. These muscles evert the foot and also help it with plantar flexion. The posterior compartment holds the large muscles of the calf, the gastrocnemius and soleus, as well as the plantaris muscle. The gastrocnemius is short and thick; it has 2 attachments, medial and lateral, and is the most visible of the calf muscles. The soleus lies underneath, and all 3 muscles attach to the Achilles tendon and aid with plantar flexion. The posterior compartment lies deep within the back of the lower leg and

Grubbs A, ed.
Taping, Wrapping, and Bracing for Athletic Trainers:
Functional Methods for Application and Fabrication (pp 63-94).
© 2017 SLACK Incorporated.

contains the tibialis posterior, flexor digitorum longus, and flexor hallucis longus and helps supinate and plantar flex the foot.

The knee joint complex consists of the femur, the tibia, the fibula, and the patella. The distal end of the femur expands and forms the convex lateral and medial condyles, which are designed to articulate with both the tibia and the patella. The articular surface of the medial condyle is longer from front to back than is the surface of the lateral condyle.[1,2] Anteriorly, the 2 condyles form a hollowed femoral groove to receive the patella.[1] The proximal end of the tibia, the tibial plateau, articulates with the condyles of the femur.[1] The tibiofemoral joint is the largest joint within the body. It is a modified hinge joint consisting of the tibia and femur with 2 degrees of freedom, flexion, and extension. The joint capsule of the knee is located between the tibia and femur. Inside the joint capsule are 2 menisci that help the tibia and femur fit uniformly. The menisci have several functions within the joint capsule that include helping to lubricate and nourish the joint, acting as shock absorbers, reducing friction in the joint, and supporting the ligaments and capsule by preventing hypertension. The patellofemoral joint is a modified plane joint in which the patella articulates with the condyles of the femur. The patella is a large sesamoid bone found within the patellar tendon. The patellar tendon is formed by the 4 quadriceps muscles coming together at the patellofemoral joint. The patella helps to improve extension and acts as a guide for gliding of the quadriceps and patellar tendons. The patella decreases friction of the quadriceps; it acts as the bony guard of the knee complex and also the pulley system of the quadriceps muscle group. The knee is supported by 4 major ligaments, 2 collateral (medial collateral and lateral collateral ligaments) and 2 cruciate (anterior cruciate and posterior cruciate ligaments). The medial collateral ligament lies medially on the tibiofemoral joint and helps to prevent valgus forces from being applied to the knee. The lateral collateral ligament lies just beneath the biceps femoris muscle and runs from the lateral epicondyle of the femur to the fibular head, preventing varus forces to the knee. The anterior cruciate ligament is composed of the anterior and the posterior bands; the 2 bands twist together and extend superiorly, posteriorly, and laterally from the tibia to the femur. The anterior cruciate ligament helps to prevent anterior movement of the tibia on the femur, lateral rotation of the tibia, and hyperextension of the knee complex. The posterior cruciate ligament extends superiorly, anteriorly, and medially from the tibia to the femur. This ligament is the strongest ligament within the knee and is that joint's primary stabilizer, resisting posterior movement of the tibia on the femur and hyperextension.

COMMON INJURIES

Lower Leg

Medial/Posterior Tibial Stress Syndrome (Shin Splints)

- The most common cause of leg pain in athletes
- Medial/posterior tibial stress syndrome is an overuse injury of the anterior/posterior tibial tendon

Mechanism of Injury

- Biomechanical deficits[2]
- Anatomical abnormalities: flattened arches or prolonged pronation[2]
- Muscle fatigue[1,2] and weakness[1]
- Training errors: training on hard surfaces or increasing load too quickly[1,2]
- Quality and condition of footwear[1,2]
- Repetitive overuse[1,2]

Common Signs and Symptoms

- Pain at the beginning of an exercise session that subsides as activity continues[1,2]
- Pain returns following completion of exercise session[1,2]
- Pain typically runs the span of the posteromedial tibial border[2]
- Painful upon palpation over medial and distal posteromedial border[2]

Knee

Anterior Cruciate Ligament Sprain/Tear

- An injury due to an external force causing an anterior displacement of the tibia relative to the femur from a noncontact-related rotational injury or hyperextension of the knee[2]
- Athletes who participate in physically demanding sports with pivoting motions like soccer, football, and basketball are more likely to injure their anterior cruciate ligaments

- Is generally considered to be one of the most serious ligament injuries to the knee[1,3]
- Female athletes are much more likely to suffer noncontact anterior cruciate ligament injuries than males[1,4-6]

Mechanism of Injury

- Torsional stress, such as pivoting or cutting in a different direction rapidly[1,2]
- Rotation of the lower leg while the foot is fixed[1]
- Anterior translation[2]
- Hyperextension of the knee[1,2]
- Direct contact to the anterior tibia in relation to the femur[1,2]
- Direct contact to the posterior femur in relation to the tibia[1,2]
- Intrinsic factors such as conditioning level, playing style, environmental conditions, and equipment[1,7]
- Strong quadriceps activation during eccentric contractions[1,8]

Common Signs and Symptoms

- Pain with possible "pop" under the kneecap[1,2]
- Diffused pain throughout the joint[2]
- Rapid effusion within the first few hours[1,2]
- Decreased range of motion with pain at end ranges[2]
- Antalgic gait[2]
- Difficulty climbing stairs[2]
- Inability to achieve full extension[2]
- Instability[1] when changing directions[2]

Posterior Cruciate Ligament

- An injury due to an external force causing a posterior displacement of the tibia relative to the femur[2]
- Quadriceps weakness can be a predisposition for posterior cruciate ligament injury[2]

Mechanism of Injury

- Posterior displacement of the tibia on the femur, often magnified when the foot is plantar flexed[1,2]

- Most at risk when the knee is flexed to 90 degrees[1]
- Hyperflexion[2]
- Hyperextension[2]

Common Signs and Symptoms

- Possible "pop" in the back of the knee[1]
- Pain within the knee joint radiating posteriorly[2]
- Pain with knee flexion past 90 degrees[2]
- Possible tenderness with palpation in the popliteal fossa[1,2]
- Antalgic gait with avoidance of full extension[2]
- No initial effusion, but may develop over time[2]
- Posterior sagging when compared bilaterally[1,2]

Lateral Knee Injury

A sprain or tear due to a traumatic incident to the lateral collateral ligament of the knee[2]

Mechanism of Injury

- Traumatic varus external force placed upon the knee[1,2]

Common Signs and Symptoms

- Pain in the lateral joint line, fibular head, or femoral condyle[2]
- Possible localized swelling over the lateral collateral ligament[1,2]
- Tenderness with palpation along the lateral collateral ligament[1,2]
- Pain and loss of motion during knee flexion and terminal extension[2]
- Lateral joint laxity[1]
- Antalgic gait due to pain[2]

Medial Knee Injury

A sprain or tear due to a traumatic incident to the medial collateral ligament of the knee[2]

Mechanism of Injury

- Traumatic valgus external force placed upon the knee[1,2]
- Less commonly due to external rotation of the tibia[1,2]

Common Signs and Symptoms

- Pain along the medial aspect of the knee[1,2]
- Tenderness along the length of the medial collateral ligament[2]
- Possible loss of function at terminal ranges of flexion and extension[1,2]

Patella Subluxation (Dislocation)

Forceful displacement of the patella often attributed to biomechanical deficits

Mechanism of Injury

- Valgus blow to the knee[2]
- Rapid change in direction with foot fixed[1,2]
- Low Q-angle, patella alta, history of patellofemoral instability,[1,2] pronated feet, and genu valgum are predisposing factors[1]

Common Signs and Symptoms

- Pain in the anterior aspect of the knee[1,2]
- Possible pain beneath the knee[2]
- If dislocated, obviously deformed[1,2]
- Effusion[1,2]
- Loss of knee function[1,2]

Patellar Tendinitis (Jumper's/Kicker's Knee)

Chronic inflammation or irritation of the patellar tendon[1]

Mechanism of Injury

- Repetitive activity involving resistive knee extension[1,2]
- Contusive force on the patella[2]
- Rapid increase in activity level[2]

Common Signs and Symptoms

- Pain at the inferior pole of the patella[1,2]
- Complain of crepitus[2]
- Pain after and/or during activity[1]
- Possibly prolonged pain after activity[1,2]
- Localized swelling[2]

- Tenderness with palpation over the patella tendon[2]
- Tendon may feel thick with crepitus present[2]

Gastrocnemius Strain (Calf Strain)

An overstretching or tearing of the muscle fibers or dynamic overload during an eccentric contraction

Mechanism of Injury

- Often injured during explosive activity such as quick starts and stops or occasional jumping[1]

Common Signs and Symptoms

- Discoloration
- Pain[1]
- Swelling[1]
- Muscle disability[1]
- "Popping" or "snapping" sound
- Possible divot in the muscle belly
- Antalgic gait
- Decreased knee range of motion

TAPE JOBS

Knee

Shin Splint Tape Job

Materials Needed

- Adhesive spray (apply prior to taping)
- Heel block
- Prewrap (optional)
- 1.5-inch white athletic tape
- 3-inch stretch tape

Step 1

Place a heel block under the leg to be taped (Figure 2-1-1).

Figure 2-1-1.

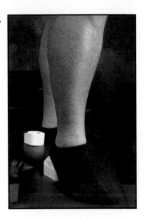

Step 2

Cover the targeted taping area with adhesive spray (Figure 2-1-2).

Figure 2-1-2.

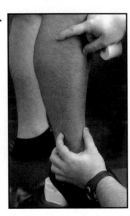

Step 3

Begin by placing an anchor around the proximal aspect of the gastrocnemius and another just proximal to the ankle (Figure 2-1-3).

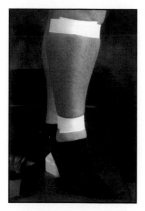

Figure 2-1-3.

Step 4

Place an anterior vertical strip from the distal to proximal anchor upon the midline of the lower leg. Then place a lateral vertical strip from the distal to proximal anchors upon the lower leg (Figure 2-1-4). (This will make a boxed area around the anterior tibialis muscle.)

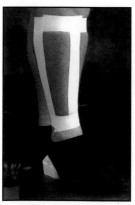

Figure 2-1-4.

Step 5

Starting at the distal anchor, place a strip of tape at the superomedial aspect of the box and pull laterally at an angle until you reach the lateral vertical strip (Figure 2-1-5).

Figure 2-1-5.

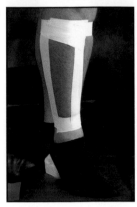

Step 6

Next, take a strip and start on the superolateral aspect of the box and pull medially at an angle until you reach the medial vertical strip. This should create a criss-cross (basketweave) pattern (Figure 2-1-6).

Figure 2-1-6.

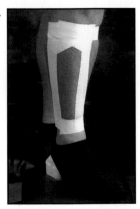

Step 7

Repeat Steps 4 and 5 until the box is completely covered. Be sure to provide significant tension throughout the basketweave pattern overlapping by half the width (Figure 2-1-7).

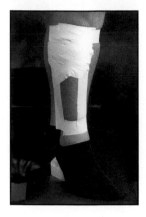

Figure 2-1-7.

Step 8

Continue with Steps 4 and 5 working distally from the proximal anchor (Figure 2-1-8).

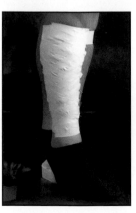

Figure 2-1-8.

Step 9

Apply another vertical strip over the previous vertical strips, securing the criss-cross strips (Figure 2-1-9).

Figure 2-1-9.

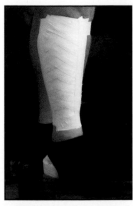

Step 10

Once the tape job is complete, elastic tape can be used to help prevent the tape job from coming loose (Figure 2-1-10).

Figure 2-1-10.

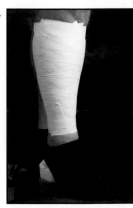

Step 11

Place another layer of anchors to secure the tape job (Figure 2-1-11).

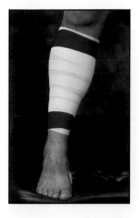

Figure 2-1-11.

Step 12

Check for capillary refill (Figure 2-1-12).

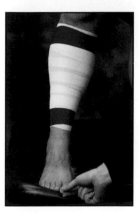

Figure 2-1-12.

Please refer to the Shin Splints tape job (Video) for further review and variation preference in performing this taping technique.

Patellar Tendon Strap (Off-the-Shelf)

Used as a method of treating patellar tendinitis to decrease pain and patellar tendon strain (Figures 2-2-1 and 2-2-2).

Figure 2-2-1.

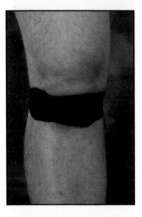

Figure 2-2-2.

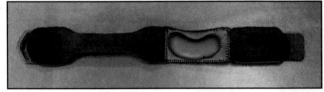

Patellar Tendon Strap (Homemade)

Materials Needed

- Prewrap

Step 1

Wrap prewrap around the knee covering a 4- to 5-inch area (Figure 2-3-1).

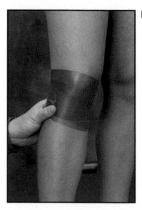

Figure 2-3-1.

Step 2

Roll the prewrap on the knee so that it forms a cord-like structure over the patellar tendon just distal to the patella (Figure 2-3-2).

Note: In order to achieve a tighter band, apply additional prewrap to create a thicker cord-like structure.

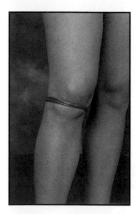

Figure 2-3-2.

Please refer to the Patellar Strap tape job (Video) for further review and variation preference in performing this taping technique.

Knee Hyperextension Tape

Materials Needed

- Adhesive spray (apply prior to taping)
- Heel block
- Stretch tape
- 1.5-inch white athletic tape
- 3-inch Elastikon

Step 1

Prepare thigh and calf region for tape by removing body hair, lotions, or gels.

Step 2

Place heel block under the athlete's foot to engage the gastrocnemius (Figure 2-4-1).

Figure 2-4-1.

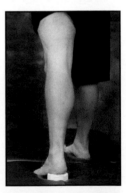

Step 3

Apply adhesive spray to targeted taping area (Figure 2-4-2).

Figure 2-4-2.

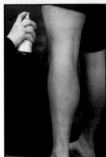

Step 4

Bend the knee to 15 degrees of flexion.

Step 5

Apply prewrap around the mid-thigh and the mid-calf (Figure 2-4-3).

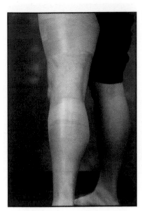

Figure 2-4-3.

Step 6

Apply 3 anchor strips to the mid-thigh with 1.5-inch white athletic tape, and 3 anchor strips to the mid-gastrocnemius with 1.5-inch white athletic tape (Figure 2-4-4).

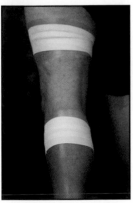

Figure 2-4-4.

Step 7

Using the Elastikon, measure the distance from the top of the mid-thigh anchor strip to the bottom of the mid-calf anchor strip with tension on the Elastikon. Repeat 3 times (Figure 2-4-5).

Figure 2-4-5.

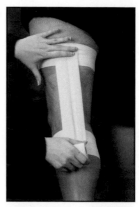

Step 8

Apply 3 strips of Elastikon in a fan-like pattern and secure the bottom of the fan to the distal anchor with 1.5-inch white athletic tape (Figure 2-4-6).

Figure 2-4-6.

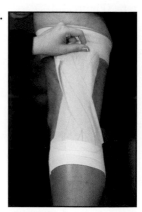

Step 9

Pulling the Elastikon proximally, attach to the proximal anchor and secure with 1.5-inch white athletic tape (Figure 2-4-7).

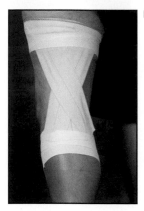

Figure 2-4-7.

Step 10

Cover with stretch tape, distal to proximal, and secure with 1.5-inch white athletic tape (Figure 2-4-8).

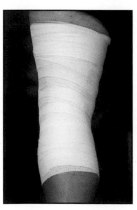

Figure 2-4-8.

Step 11

Check for capillary refill (Figure 2-4-9).

Figure 2-4-9.

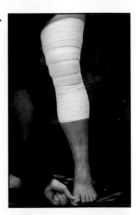

Please refer to the Knee Hyperextension tape job (Video) for further review and variation preference in performing this taping technique.

Knee Stabilization Tape

Materials Needed

- Adhesive spray (apply prior to taping)
- Prewrap
- 1.5-inch white tape
- 2-inch block or wedge
- 2-inch Elastikon
- 3-inch PowerFlex (Andover Healthcare, Inc)

Step 1

Place a 2-inch block or wedge under the heel of the foot. This will provide flexion at the knee (Figure 2-5-1).

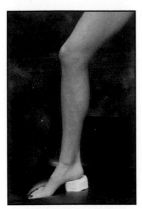

Figure 2-5-1.

Step 2

Apply adhesive spray to targeted taping area and apply prewrap if desired (Figure 2-5-2).

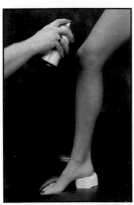

Figure 2-5-2.

Step 3

Begin by placing 3 anchor strips on the proximal aspect of the gastrocnemius and 3 anchor strips on the distal aspect of the thigh (Figure 2-5-3).

Figure 2-5-3.

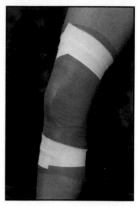

Step 4

Using 2-inch Elastikon tape, take 2 strips and create an X shape, crossing the lateral knee joint line with moderate tension. The first strip begins on the posterior aspect of the proximal anchor, crosses the joint line, and ends on the anterior portion of distal anchor. The second strip begins on the anterior portion of the proximal anchor and ends on the posterior portion of the distal anchor (Figure 2-5-4).

Figure 2-5-4.

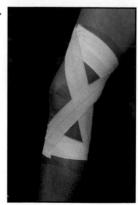

Step 5

Place an additional vertical strip of Elastikon over the existing X with moderate tension. Then repeat Steps 3 and 4 again (Figure 2-5-5).

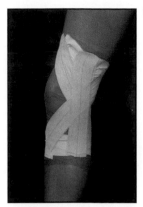

Figure 2-5-5.

Step 6

Cover the ends of the Elastikon with proximal and distal anchor strips (Figure 2-5-6).

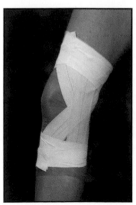

Figure 2-5-6.

Step 7

Check for capillary refill (Figure 2-5-7).

Note: This tape job can also be repeated on the lateral aspect of the knee to stabilize the knee.

Figure 2-5-7.

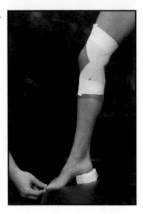

Please refer to the Knee Stabilization tape job (Video) for further review and variation preference in performing this taping technique.

Hinged Brace

Materials Needed

- Appropriate-sized knee brace
- **Note:** Appropriate type of knee brace, realizing that some are basically a hinge mechanism and others are a sleeve-type with hinges attached
- Tape measure

Step 1

Begin by measuring the girth of the knee. Do this by measuring the circumference of the leg approximately 6 inches above and below the patella (Figures 2-6-1A and B).

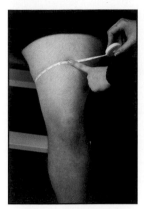

Figure 2-6-1A.

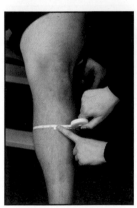

Figure 2-6-1B.

Step 2

Once you have the measurements, select the appropriate-sized brace based on the manufacturer's sizing chart.

Step 3

Loosen straps and align with the proper knee (left or right; Figure 2-6-2).

Figure 2-6-2.

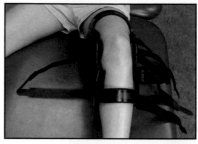

Step 4

Start securing the brace based on the manufacturer's recommendations for the best outcome (Figure 2-6-3).

Figure 2-6-3.

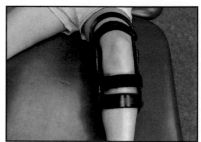

Derotation Brace

Materials Needed

- Derotation brace
- Tape measure

Step 1

Begin by measuring the girth of the knee. Do this by measuring the circumference of the leg approximately 6 inches above and below the patella (Figures 2-7-1A and B).

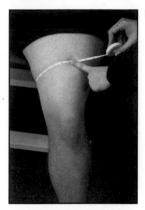

Figure 2-7-1A.

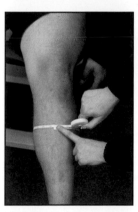

Figure 2-7-1B.

Step 2

Once you have the measurements, select the appropriate-sized brace based on the manufacturer's sizing chart.

Step 3

Dry-run align with medial and lateral aspect of the knee, properly fitting the appropriate-sized condylar padding (Figure 2-7-2).

Figure 2-7-2. (Reprinted with permission from Breg, Inc.)

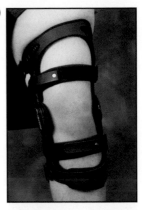

Step 4

Align medial and lateral hinges appropriately with the knee (Figure 2-7-3).

Figure 2-7-3. (Reprinted with permission from Breg, Inc.)

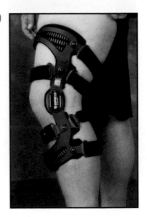

Knee Stabilizing Brace

Materials Needed

- Compression sleeve (neoprene, stockinette, or other material to cushion)
- Lateral stabilizing brace
- Tape measure

Step 1

Begin by measuring the girth of the knee. Do this by measuring the circumference of the leg approximately 6 inches above and below the patella (Figures 2-8-1A and B).

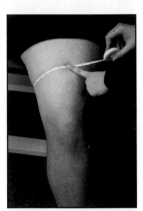

Figure 2-8-1A.

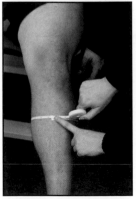

Figure 2-8-1B.

Step 2

Once you have the measurements, select the appropriate-sized brace based upon the manufacturer's sizing chart.

Step 3

Align the lateral stabilizer with the appropriate knee, and secure based upon the manufacturer's recommendations (Figures 2-8-2A and B).

Figure 2-8-2A.

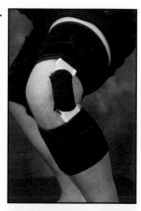

Figure 2-8-2B.

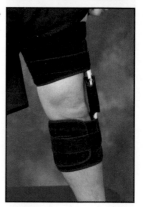

Knee Compression Wrap/Sleeve

Use of a compression sleeve or compression wrap is multipurpose, such as under prophylactic bracing as a buffer between the individual's skin and the brace. Another use is postinjury in the acute phase to help control swelling.

Materials Needed

- Ace wrap (3M Company)

Step 1

Starting distal to the knee, begin wrapping around the lower leg with moderate tension working up with every time around overlapping by half to two-thirds the width of the wrap. Continue until the wrap ends and is up to the mid-thigh. Check for capillary refill (Figure 2-9-1).

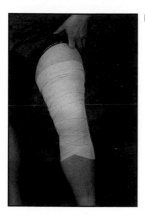

Figure 2-9-1.

Please refer to the Knee Compression Sleeve tape job (Video) for further review and variation preference in performing this taping technique.

REFERENCES

1. Prentice WE. *Arnheim's Principles of Athletic Training: A Competency-Based Approach.* 14th ed. New York, NY: McGraw-Hill; 2010.
2. Starkey C, Brown SD. *Examination of Orthopedic and Athletic Injuries.* 4th ed. Philadelphia, PA: FA Davis Co; 2015.
3. Mangine RE, Kremchek TE. Evaluation-based protocol of the anterior cruciate ligament. *J Sport Rehabil.* 1997;6:157-181.
4. Arendt EA, Agel J, Dick R. Anterior cruciate ligament injury patterns among collegiate men and women. *J Athl Train.* 1999;34(2):86-92.

5. Ireland ML. Anterior cruciate ligament injury in female athletes: epidemiology. *J Athl Train.* 1999;34(2):150-154.
6. Cimino F, Volk BS, Setter D. Anterior cruciate ligament injury: diagnosis, management, and prevention. *Am Fam Physician.* 2010;82(8):917-922.
7. Moul JL. Differences in selected predictors of anterior cruciate ligament tears between male and female NCAA division I collegiate basketball players. *J Athl Train.* 1998;33(2):118-121.
8. Rosene JM, Fogarty TD. Anterior tibial translation in collegiate athletes with normal anterior cruciate ligament integrity. *J Athl Train.* 1999;34(2):93-98.

BIBLIOGRAPHY

Craig DI. Medial tibial stress syndrome: evidence-based prevention. *J Athl Train.* 2008;43(3):316-318.

Galbraith RM, Lavallee ME. Medial tibial stress syndrome: conservative treatment options. *Curr Rev Musculoskelet Med.* 2009;2(3):127-133.

Kortebein PM, Kaufman KR, Basford JR, Stuart MJ. Medial tibial stress syndrome. *Med Sci Sports Exerc.* 2000;32(3 suppl):S27-S33.

Moen MH, Tol JL, Weir A, Steunebrink M, De Winter TC. Medial tibial stress syndrome. *Sports Med.* 2009;39(7):523-546.

Mubarak SJ, Gould RN, Lee YF, Schmidt DA, Hargens AR. The medial tibial stress syndrome. A cause of shin splints. *Am J Sports Med.* 1982;10(4):201-205.

Please see videos on the accompanying website at
www.healio.com/books/tapingAT

3

Hip and Thigh

INTRODUCTION AND ANATOMY

The thigh, hip, and pelvis have relatively lower incidences of injury when compared to the knee and ankle, but can nevertheless be subject to considerable trauma from a variety of activities.[1] The part of the leg between the hip and the knee, commonly referred to as the thigh, is supported by the femur, which is the longest and strongest bone in the body, designed to permit maximum mobility while providing support during locomotion.[1]

The hip joint is a multiaxial ball-and-socket joint and one of the largest and most stable joints in the body. Its stability is due to the deep articulation of the femoral head in the acetabulum of the hip. Within the acetabulum, as within the shoulder socket, lies a ring of fibrocartilage called the labrum. This structure deepens the articulation between the acetabulum and femoral head, and by securing the latter, helps to stabilize the hip joint.

The hip is supported by 3 strong ligaments: the iliofemoral, the ischiofemoral, and the pubofemoral. The iliofemoral ligament is considered the strongest ligament in the body: it prevents excessive extension and helps maintain upright posture of the hip. The ischiofemoral ligament is the weakest of the 3 hip ligaments. Its role is to help stabilize the hip in extension, while the role of the pubofemoral ligament is to limit extension and prevent excessive abduction of the femur.

Grubbs A, ed.
*Taping, Wrapping, and Bracing for Athletic Trainers:
Functional Methods for Application and Fabrication* (pp 95-115).
© 2017 SLACK Incorporated.

The gluteals are the 3 muscles of the buttocks: the gluteus maximus, gluteus minimus, and gluteus medius. These attach to the back of the pelvis and insert into the greater trochanter of the femur.

The 4 quadriceps muscles—vastus lateralis, vastus medialis, vastus intermedius, and rectus femoris—are located anterior to the femur. They converge to form the patellar tendon, which inserts on the tibial tuberosity. The rectus femoris originates at the front of the ileum; the 3 other quads originate near or just below the greater trochanter of the femur.

The primary hip flexor muscle is the iliopsoas. Its 3 parts attach to the lower portion of the spine and pelvis, then cross the joint, and insert into the lesser trochanter of the femur.

The muscles that originate in the posterior thigh are called the hamstrings and include the semitendinosus, semimembranosus, and biceps femoris muscles. All 3 attach to the lowest part of the pelvis.

Finally, the groin or adductor muscles are fan-like muscles in the upper thigh that pull the legs together when they contract. They also help stabilize the hip joint. The adductors run from the pelvis to the femur, attach to the pubis, and run down the inside of the thigh. As their name suggests, these muscles help with adduction of the hip joint. The adductors also assist in outward and inward rotation, flexion, and extension.

COMMON INJURIES

Hip

Groin Injury (Strain)

Mechanism of Injury

- Groin strain or tear is a result of overloading the adductor muscle group
- Athletes who cut or change direction rapidly during activity are more susceptible to groin injuries

Common Signs and Symptoms

- Pain and tenderness in the groin and the inside of the thigh
- Pain when bringing the legs together
- Pain when raising the knee
- A popping or snapping sensation during the motion, followed by severe pain

Iliopsoas Injury (Strain)

Mechanism of Injury

- Hip hyperextension[2]
- Resisted hip flexion[2]

Common Signs and Symptoms

- Painful active hip flexion[2]
- Painful passive hip extension[2]
- Pain when climbing stairs[2]
- Decreased range of motion[2]
- Localized pain at the attachment site[2]
- Popping or snapping sensation[2]
- Possible palpable divot[2]
- Edema or ecchymosis[2]
- Antalgic gait[2]
- Possible discoloration

Thigh

Hamstring Injury (Strain/Rupture)

Mechanism of Injury

- Dynamic overload; eccentric contraction[2]
- Tensile force; overstretching the muscle[2]
- Most commonly involves the long head of the biceps femoris[2]

Common Signs and Symptoms

- Painful active knee flexion and hip extension with an extended knee[2]
- Painful passive knee extension and hip flexion[2]
- Decreased range of motion[2]
- Localizcd pain at the attachment site[2]
- Popping or snapping sensation[2]
- Possible palpable divot[2]
- Edema or ecchymosis[2]

- Antalgic gait[2]
- Possible discoloration

Iliotibial Band Syndrome

Mechanism of Injury

- One of the more common overuse injuries of the lower extremity
- It can be attributed to training habits, anatomical abnormalities, or muscular imbalances (eg, running on canted surfaces such as a road or indoor track, high or low arches, supination, or weak hip muscles)

Common Signs and Symptoms

- Knee pain from the inflamed iliotibial band snapping over the femoral condyle
- Pain with flexion
- Tenderness upon palpation of the iliotibial band insertion or bursae
- Possible muscular imbalance in the quadriceps

Rectus Femoris Injury (Strain/Rupture)

Mechanism of Injury

- Hyperextension of the hip and flexion of the knee[2]
- Dynamic overload; isometric contraction[2]

Common Signs and Symptoms

- Pain with active hip flexion and knee extension[2]
- Pain with passive hip extension and knee flexion[2]
- Pain when climbing stairs[2]
- Decreased range of motion[2]
- Localized pain at the attachment site[2]
- Popping or snapping sensation[2]
- Possible palpable divot[2]
- Edema or ecchymosis[2]
- Antalgic gait[2]
- Possible discoloration

Vastus Medialis/Lateralis/Intermedius Injury (Strain/Rupture)

Mechanism of Injury

- Hyperflexion of the knee[2]
- Dynamic overload; resisted knee extension[2]

Common Signs and Symptoms

- Pain with active knee extension with a flexed knee[2]
- Pain with passive knee flexion[2]
- Pain when climbing stairs[2]
- Decreased range of motion[2]
- Localized pain at the attachment site[2]
- Popping or snapping sensation[2]
- Possible palpable divot[2]
- Edema or ecchymosis[2]
- Antalgic gait[2]
- Possible discoloration

TAPE JOBS

Hip

Compression Wraps

Hamstring Compression Wrap

Materials Needed

- Ace wrap (6-inch single or double)
- Adhesive spray (apply prior to taping)
- 1.5-inch white athletic tape or elastic stretch tape
- 2-inch block or wedge

Step 1

Apply adhesive spray to targeted taping area (Figure 3-1-1).

Figure 3-1-1.

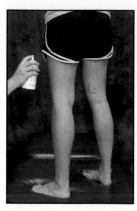

Step 2

Place a 2-inch block or wedge under the heel of the foot. This will provide flexion at the hip prior to wrapping (Figure 3-1-2).

Figure 3-1-2.

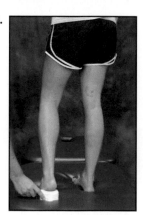

Step 3

Start wrapping the rolled Ace wrap at the distal, posterior aspect of the hamstring with moderate tension (Figure 3-1-3).

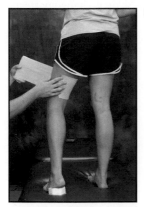

Figure 3-1-3.

Step 4

Once the Ace wrap reaches the starting point, begin pulling superiorly around the leg (Figure 3-1-4).

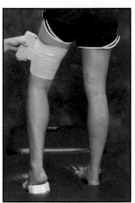

Figure 3-1-4.

Step 5

Overlapping three-quarters to half the width of the Ace wrap already laid to the skin, alternate pulling the wrap superiorly and inferiorly around the leg (Figure 3-1-5).

Note: This should begin to resemble a criss-cross X- or V-shaped pattern.

Figure 3-1-5.

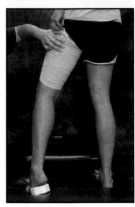

Step 6

Repeat until the entire hamstring is covered and the Ace wrap is unrolled.

Step 7

Using 1.5-inch white athletic tape or elastic stretch tape, secure the Ace wrap to the leg (Figure 3-1-6).

Figure 3-1-6.

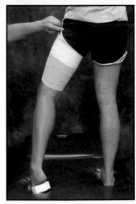

Step 8

Check for capillary refill (Figure 3-1-7).

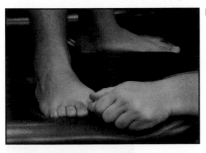

Figure 3-1-7.

Please refer to the Hamstring Compression Wrap tape job (Video) for further review and variation preference in performing this taping technique.

Thigh Compression Wrap

Materials Needed

- Ace wrap (6-inch single or double)
- Adhesive spray (apply prior to taping)
- 1.5-inch white athletic tape or elastic stretch tape
- 2-inch block or wedge

Step 1

Apply adhesive spray to targeted wrapping area (Figure 3-2-1).

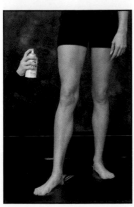

Figure 3-2-1.

Step 2

Place a 2-inch block or wedge under the heel of the foot. This will provide flexion at the hip prior to wrapping (Figure 3-2-2).

Figure 3-2-2.

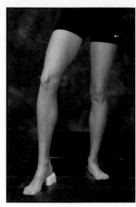

Step 3

Start wrapping the rolled Ace wrap at the distal, anterior aspect of the quadriceps with moderate tension (Figure 3-2-3).

Figure 3-2-3.

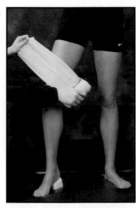

Step 4

Once the Ace wrap reaches the starting point, begin pulling superiorly around the leg (Figure 3-2-4).

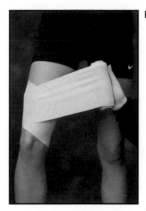

Figure 3-2-4.

Step 5

Overlapping three-quarters to half the width of the Ace wrap already laid to the skin, alternate pulling the wrap superiorly and inferiorly around the leg (Figure 3-2-5).

Note: This should begin to resemble a criss-cross X- or V-shaped pattern.

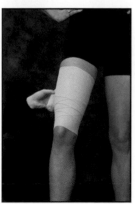

Figure 3-2-5.

Step 6

Repeat until the entire quadriceps is covered and the Ace wrap is unrolled (Figure 3-2-6).

Figure 3-2-6.

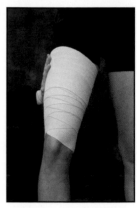

Step 7

Using 1.5-inch white athletic tape or elastic stretch tape, secure the Ace wrap to the leg (Figure 3-2-7).

Figure 3-2-7.

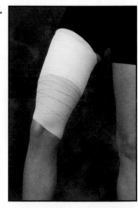

Step 8

Check for capillary refill (Figure 3-2-8).

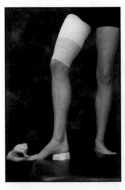

Figure 3-2-8.

Please refer to the Thigh Compression Wrap tape job (Video) for further review and variation preference in performing this taping technique.

Hip Adduction Groin

Materials Needed

- Ace wrap (6-inch double)
- 1.5-inch white athletic tape or elastic stretch tape
- 2-inch block or wedge

Step 1

Place a 2-inch block or wedge under the heel of the foot. This will provide flexion at the hip prior to wrapping. Also, the athlete should internally rotate his or her hip and maintain this position (Figure 3-3-1).

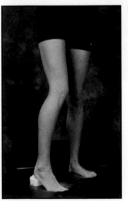

Figure 3-3-1.

Step 2

Starting at the distal aspect of the quadriceps muscle belly, apply tension superolaterally until reaching the posterior aspect of the leg (Figure 3-3-2).

Figure 3-3-2.

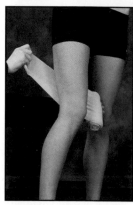

Step 3

Having reached the posterior aspect, begin to pull inferomedially until reaching the starting point (Figure 3-3-3).

Figure 3-3-3.

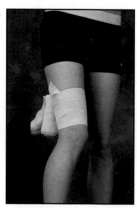

Step 4

Overlapping three-quarters to half the width of the Ace wrap already laid to the skin, pull the wrap around the anterior aspect of the leg, creating an X or V pattern working superiorly with every time around (Figure 3-3-4).

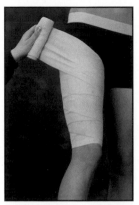

Figure 3-3-4.

Step 5

When you reach the top of the thigh, pass the wrap posteriorly over the hip at the iliac crest, opposite the thigh being wrapped, around the lateral aspect of the hip, and return to the proximal lateral aspect of the thigh (Figure 3-3-5).

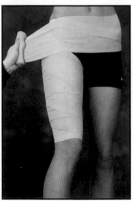

Figure 3-3-5.

Step 6

Work your way back inferomedially around the thigh once and back superolaterally to the starting point on the lateral hip. Repeat Steps 5 and 6 until you run out of wrap (Figure 3-3-6).

Note: This should begin to resemble a criss-cross X- or V-shaped pattern.

Figure 3-3-6.

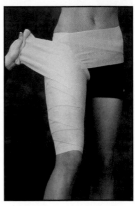

Step 7

Cover the end of the Ace wrap with stretch tape to close the wrap securely (Figure 3-3-7).

Figure 3-3-7.

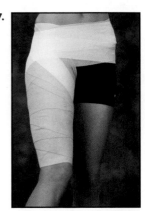

Step 8

Check for capillary refill (Figure 3-3-8).

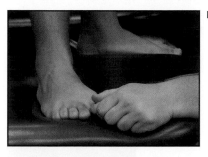

Figure 3-3-8.

Please refer to the Hip Adduction Groin tape job (Video) for further review and variation preference in performing this taping technique.

Hip Abduction Flexor

Materials Needed

- Ace wrap (6-inch double)
- 1.5-inch white athletic tape or elastic stretch tape
- 2-inch block or wedge

Step 1

Place a 2-inch block or wedge under the heel of the foot, and have the athlete rotate his or her hip internally. This will provide flexion at the hip prior to wrapping. The athlete should maintain this position throughout the process (Figure 3-4-1).

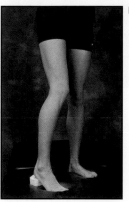

Figure 3-4-1.

Step 2

Starting at the distal aspect of the quadriceps muscle belly, apply tension medially until reaching the posterior aspect of the leg (Figure 3-4-2).

Figure 3-4-2.

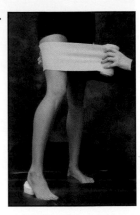

Step 3

Once the posterior aspect has been reached, begin pulling laterally until reaching the starting point (Figure 3-4-3).

Figure 3-4-3.

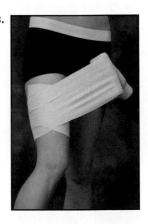

Step 4

Overlapping three-quarters to half the width of the Ace wrap already laid to the skin, pull the wrap with moderate tension around the leg, creating an X or V pattern (Figure 3-4-4).

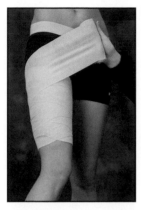

Figure 3-4-4.

Step 5

When you reach the top of the thigh and come around the posterior aspect, pass the wrap anteriorly over the iliac crest, opposite the thigh being wrapped, around the lateral aspect of the hip, and return to the proximal lateral aspect of the thigh, which is the starting point (Figure 3-4-5).

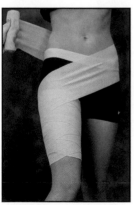

Figure 3-4-5.

Step 6

Wrap inferomedially around the medial leg and back superolaterally until reaching the starting point on the lateral hip. Repeat Steps 5 and 6 until you run out of wrap (Figure 3-4-6).

Note: This should begin to resemble a criss-cross X- or V-shaped pattern.

Figure 3-4-6.

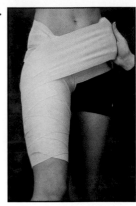

Step 7

Cover the end of the Ace wrap with stretch tape to close the wrap securely (Figure 3-4-7).

Figure 3-4-7.

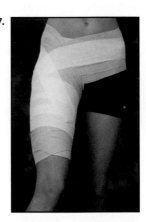

Step 8

Check for capillary refill (Figure 3-4-8).

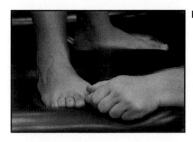

Figure 3-4-8.

Please refer to the Hip Abduction Flexors tape job (Video) for further review and variation preference in performing this taping technique.

McDavid Cross Compression Shorts

Materials Needed

- Appropriate-sized compression shorts (Figure 3-5-1)
- Size chart

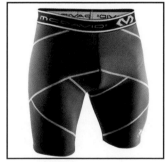

Figure 3-5-1. (Reprinted with permission from United Sports Brands.)

REFERENCES

1. Prentice WE. *Arnheim's Principles of Athletic Training: A Competency-Based Approach.* 14th ed. New York, NY: McGraw-Hill; 2010.
2. Starkey C, Brown SD. *Examination of Orthopedic and Athletic Injuries.* 4th ed. Philadelphia, PA: FA Davis Co; 2015.

Please see videos on the accompanying website at
www.healio.com/books/tapingAT

4

Shoulder and Elbow

INTRODUCTION AND ANATOMY

The shoulder consists of 4 major joints: the glenohumeral, acromioclavicular, sternoclavicular, and scapulothoracic. The glenohumeral joint is a multiaxial, ball-and-socket joint. Because the articulations of the humerus are weak, the shoulder relies more on the surrounding muscles and ligaments for stability and support. The humeral head articulates with the glenoid fossa. The labrum, which is a ring of fibrocartilage, encapsulates the glenoid fossa and helps support the humeral head more securely. The primary ligaments of the glenohumeral joint are the superior, middle, and inferior glenohumeral ligaments. The acromioclavicular joint is a synovial joint formed by the articulation of the acromion process of the scapula and the lateral end of the clavicle. The sternoclavicular joint acts like the acromioclavicular joint by helping to increase the humeral range of motion within the glenoid fossa. Lastly, the scapulothoracic joint, which is an articulating joint, has an important role within the shoulder complex, enabling it to function precisely during anatomical movements. The scapulothoracic joint consists of the scapula and the muscles of the posterior chest wall. It is important that the musculature surrounding the scapula has maximum strength in order to help prevent chronic issues, such as scapular winging, which in turn will help strengthen the rotator cuff muscles. Four main muscles make-up the rotator cuff: the supraspinatus, infraspinatus, teres

Grubbs A, ed.
Taping, Wrapping, and Bracing for Athletic Trainers:
Functional Methods for Application and Fabrication (pp 117-133).
© 2017 SLACK Incorporated.

minor, and subscapularis. (An easy way to remember them is with the acronym "SITS.") The muscles of the rotator cuff play a key role in moving the shoulder through its full range of motion.

The elbow's primary role is to help position the hand so it can perform a desired function. The elbow consists of the articulations of the ulnohumeral, radiohumeral, and superior radioulnar joints. The ulnohumeral joint is located between the trochlea of the humerus and trochlear notch of the ulna and is classified as a hinge joint. The radiohumeral joint is a hinge joint located between the capitulum of the humerus and the head of the radius. The ulnohumeral and radiohumeral joints are supported medially by the ulnar collateral ligament and laterally by the radial collateral ligament. Lastly, the superior radioulnar joint is classified as a pivot joint and allows for the pronation and supination of the forearm. The annular ligament helps to strengthen the articulation of the radius and ulna. The cubital fossa is triangular in shape and thus has 3 sides: the lateral side (the medial border of the brachioradialis muscle), the medial side (the lateral border of the pronator teres muscle), and the superior side (an imaginary line between the epicondyles of the humerus).

COMMON INJURIES

Shoulder

Acromioclavicular Sprain

Stretching or tearing of the acromioclavicular ligament or coracoclavicular ligaments

Mechanism of Injury

- Falling on an outstretched hand[1,2]
- Falling directly on the tip of the shoulder, landing on an outstretched arm[1,2]

Common Signs and Symptoms

- Possible displacement of the clavicle[1,2]
- Point tenderness over the acromioclavicular joint[1,2]
- Referred pain to the upper trapezius or upper scapula[1]
- Possible step-off deformity (also known as piano key sign)[1]

- Decreased range of motion in abduction[2] and flexion
- Pain with elevation, protraction, and retraction of the scapula[1]

Rotator Cuff Tendinopathy

Acute or chronic inflammation of the musculature associated with the rotator cuff[1]

Mechanism of Injury

- Acute
- Dynamic overloading of the tendon[1]
- Insidious
- Chronic impingement[1]
- Single traumatic episode may cause final rupture of a weakened tendon[1]
- Degenerative change in the tissue[1]
- Repetitive overhead motion[1]

Common Signs and Symptoms

- Deep pain within the shoulder beneath the acromion process[1]
- Referred pain into the lateral arm[1]
- Possible clicking during certain glenohumeral motions[1]
- Tenderness in the subacromial space and at the insertion of the supraspinatus tendon into the greater tuberosity[1]
- Painful active range of motion with elevation, especially in abduction[1]
- Decreased strength with abduction, internal rotation, external rotation, and elevation in scaption[1]

Elbow

Hyperextension

Forceful hyperextension of the elbow

Mechanism of Injury

- Falling on an outstretched hand with the elbow locked in extension
- Blunt force trauma

Common Signs and Symptoms

- Pain in the cubital fossa
- Pain in the posterior elbow
- Inflammation of the bursa and/or surrounding structures
- Discoloration around the posterior elbow
- Decreased range of motion, flexion, and extension
- Feeling of weakness or instability
- Possible fracture to the humerus and/or ulna

Medial Epicondylitis (Golfer's Elbow)

Irritation or inflammation of wrist flexors often due to repetitive trauma[1,2]

Mechanism of Injury

- Repetitive, forceful flexion or pronation of the wrist[1,2]
- Repetitive eccentric loading of the medial elbow muscles[1]

Common Signs and Symptoms

- Pain at the medial epicondyle[2] and the proximal portion of the wrist flexor and pronator muscles[1]
- Inflammation over the medial epicondyle[1,2]
- Painful active range of motion with wrist flexion and wrist extension due to stretching of involved muscles[1,2]
- Decreased strength with wrist flexors and pronators[1]

Lateral Epicondylitis (Tennis Elbow)

Irritation or repetitive stresses at the lateral epicondyle at the common attachment site of the wrist extensor group[1,2]

Mechanism of Injury

- Overuse involving repetitive, forceful wrist extension[1]
- Repetitive eccentric loading of the wrist extensors[1,2]

Common Signs and Symptoms

- Inflammation over the lateral epicondyle[1]
- Pain[2] and possible crepitus over the lateral epicondyle and common wrist extensor tendon[1]

- Limited active and passive range of motion with wrist flexion, radial deviation, elbow extension, and pronation[1,2]
- Pain or weakness with gripping[1]

TAPE JOBS

Shoulder and Elbow

Shoulder Spica

Materials Needed

- Elastic adhesive tape or 1.5-inch white athletic tape
- 4- to 6-inch Ace wrap (single or double)

Step 1

Have the patient place the hand of the shoulder to be wrapped on his or her hip. Place the opposite arm away from the body (Figure 4-1-1).

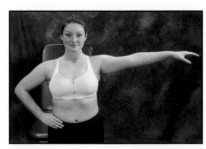

Figure 4-1-1.

Step 2

Then start the Ace wrap on the lateral mid-shaft of the humerus, placing the Ace wrap to the skin and pulling superolaterally. Once reaching the posterior aspect of the humerus, change the angle of the pull inferomedially until reaching the starting point. Overlapping three-quarters to half the width of the Ace wrap already laid to the skin, work your way proximally until you reach the acromion (Figure 4-1-2).

Figure 4-1-2.

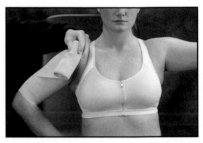

Step 3

Just before you reach the level of the acromion, begin to pass the wrap anteriorly around the body, under the other shoulder, across the back, and return to the anterior aspect of the acromion (Figure 4-1-3).

Figure 4-1-3.

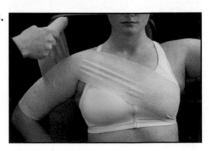

Step 4

Once returning to the starting point, the acromion, continue to pull laterally and pass around the posterior aspect of the humerus. Overlapping three-quarters to half the width of the Ace wrap already laid to the skin, continue until the Ace wrap ends (Figure 4-1-4).

Note: This should resemble a criss-cross X- or V-shaped pattern.

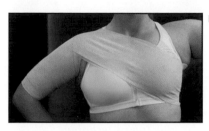

Figure 4-1-4.

Step 5

Then use 1.5-inch white athletic tape or elastic adhesive tape to secure the spica (Figure 4-1-5).

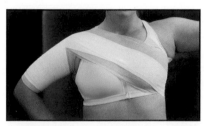

Figure 4-1-5.

Step 6

Test restrictions until you have achieved proper range of motion (Figure 4-1-6).

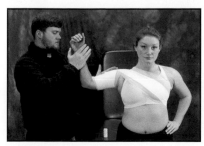

Figure 4-1-6.

Step 7

Check for capillary refill (Figure 4-1-7).

Figure 4-1-7.

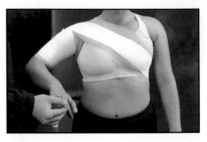

Please refer to the Shoulder Spica tape job (Video) for further review and variation preference in performing this taping technique.

Acromioclavicular Pad

Materials Needed

- Ace wrap
- Adhesive spray (apply prior to taping)
- Foam or felt

Step 1

Apply adhesive spray to pad area (Figure 4-2-1).

Figure 4-2-1.

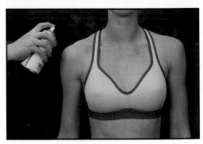

Step 2

Using felt or foam material, cut a pad that will cover the acromioclavicular joint (Figure 4-2-2).

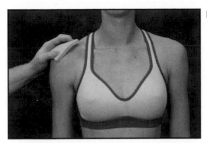

Figure 4-2-2.

Step 3

Once the proper sized pad has been cut, secure the pad to the acromioclavicular joint with Ace wrap using the shoulder spica technique (Figure 4-2-3).

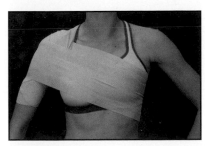

Figure 4-2-3.

Elbow Hyperextension

Materials Needed

- Adhesive spray (apply prior to taping)
- Prewrap (optional)
- 1.5-inch white athletic tape
- 2- to 3-inch Elastikon

Step 1

Apply adhesive spray to targeted taping area. Apply prewrap from the proximal to distal aspects of the elbow (Figure 4-3-1).

Figure 4-3-1.

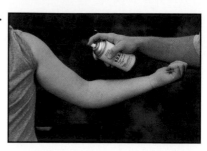

Step 2

With the athlete contracting his or her biceps, begin by applying anchor strips around the belly of the biceps (Figure 4-3-2).

Figure 4-3-2.

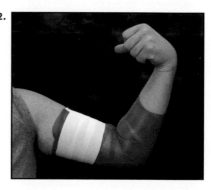

Step 3

With the athlete flexing the forearm, apply another set of anchor strips around the proximal forearm (Figure 4-3-3).

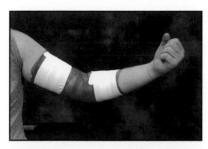

Figure 4-3-3.

Step 4

Using Elastikon, split each end, creating a Y shape, to allow secure attachment to the anchor strips (Figure 4-3-4).

Note: A fan made with 1.5-inch white athletic tape can be used as a substitute for Elastikon.

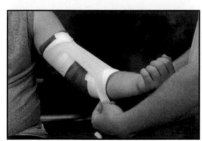

Figure 4-3-4.

Step 5

Have the athlete extend the elbow until pain is present. Flex the athlete's elbow slightly in order to stay within a pain-free range of motion (Figure 4-3-5).

Figure 4-3-5.

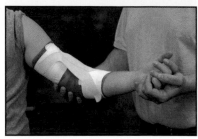

Step 6

Attach Elastikon to the bicep anchor. Apply tension to the Elastikon and attach to the forearm anchor (Figure 4-3-6).

Figure 4-3-6.

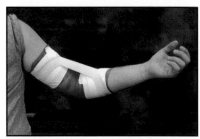

Step 7

Apply a second Elastikon band to increase strength (Figure 4-3-7).

Figure 4-3-7.

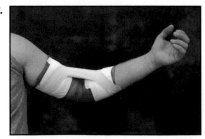

Step 8

Secure with anchors on both ends (Figure 4-3-8).

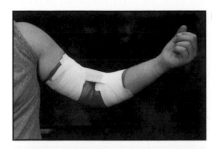

Figure 4-3-8.

Step 9

Cover with stretch tape to close the tape job (Figure 4-3-9).

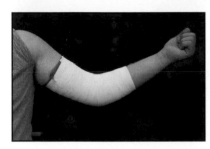

Figure 4-3-9.

Step 10

Check for capillary refill (Figure 4-3-10).

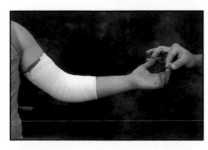

Figure 4-3-10.

Please refer to the Elbow Hyperextension tape job (Video) for further review and variation preference in performing this taping technique.

Elbow Compression Sleeve

An elbow compression sleeve can be used for a multitude of pathologies. Oftentimes, elbow compression sleeves are used for inflammation, bursitis, and general support or stability. While application may be simple, be sure the desired therapeutic effect is being achieved.

Materials Needed

- Appropriate-sized elbow compression sleeve

Step 1

Apply the appropriate-sized elbow compression sleeve (Figure 4-4-1).

Figure 4-4-1.

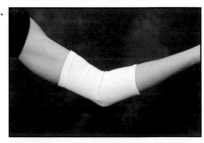

Step 2

Check for capillary refill.

Note: If the compression sleeve has straps, 1.5-inch white athletic tape or stretch tape can be used to secure.

Please refer to the Elbow Compression Sleeve tape job (Video) for further review and variation preference in performing this taping technique.

Sully Brace

A Sully brace is often used to prevent the shoulder from moving into an undesirable range of motion (Figures 4-5-1 and 4-5-2). Typically, this brace is used to assist with anterior instabilities, multidirectional instabilities, inferior instabilities, posterior instabilities, rotator cuff deceleration, and muscle strains. Start with the athlete's arm in the hands-on-hips position for the majority of the wraps. Modify the starting position as desired to increase or decrease stabilization or assistance. Keep the straps taut during application and adjust tension levels as necessary. Move the fixed hook and loop end of the strap closer to the elbow when higher levels of stabilization are desired. Move the fixed hook and loop end of the strap closer to the shoulder for lighter support or to allow increased mobility. Finally, be creative; the

Sully can be custom fit for each application. Tailor the wrapping process to the needs of the athlete.

Materials Needed

- Appropriate-sized Sully brace
- Associated straps (2 to 3)

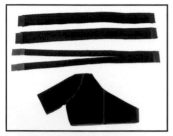

Figure 4-5-1. (Reprinted with permission from DJO Global.)

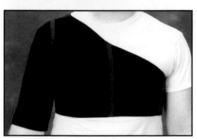

Figure 4-5-2. (Reprinted with permission from DJO Global.)

DonJoy Shoulder Stabilizer

A DonJoy Shoulder Stabilizer brace is often used to prevent the shoulder from moving into an undesirable range of motion. Typically, this brace is used to prevent anterior dislocations/subluxations and excessive abduction or horizontal abduction, which can often place the shoulder in a compromised position. It may also be used to limit extension, protraction, retraction, and elevation. The shoulder brace is also effective in supporting acromioclavicular separations. If the joint is still tender, a donut or protective pad can be placed under the brace. Tighten the acromioclavicular strap by adjusting the strap through the front and back D rings. The long or medium auxiliary straps can also be threaded through the loops over the acromioclavicular joint and attached to the hook and loop at the front and back of the brace. This type of stabilization brace can be utilized for the following types of athletes:

- Offensive linemen
- Defensive linemen
- Linebacker

Materials Needed

- Appropriate-sized DonJoy Shoulder Stabilizer

Step 1

Apply the brace over the injured shoulder. Grasp one end of the brace at the bottom and pull over the hook and loop closure, making sure to close the bottom tighter than the top. The fit should be snug but should not restrict breathing (Figure 4-6-1).

Figure 4-6-1. (Reprinted with permission from DJO Global.)

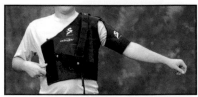

Step 2

Secure the hook and loop strap through the D ring to lock in the side closure. Attach the hook and loop closures at the biceps, trying to get as tight a fit as possible; this will minimize any rotation within (Figure 4-6-2).

Figure 4-6-2. (Reprinted with permission from DJO Global.)

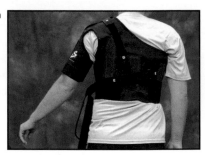

Step 3

To achieve simple abduction control, after applying the brace, attach the glenohumeral straps to the biceps cuff with the stitching attaching the front and back straps. This positioning is very important (Figure 4-6-3).

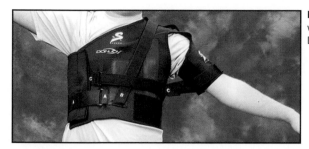

Figure 4-6-3. (Reprinted with permission from DJO Global.)

Step 4

Simply tighten or loosen the straps through the D rings and hook and loop to achieve the desired range of motion and abduction control (Figure 4-6-4).

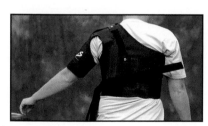

Figure 4-6-4. (Reprinted with permission from DJO Global.)

REFERENCES

1. Starkey C, Brown SD. *Examination of Orthopedic and Athletic Injuries.* 4th ed. Philadelphia, PA: FA Davis Co; 2015.
2. Prentice WE. *Arnheim's Principles of Athletic Training: A Competency-Based Approach.* 14th ed. New York, NY: McGraw-Hill; 2010.

Please see videos on the accompanying website at
www.healio.com/books/tapingAT

5

Forearm, Wrist, and Fingers

INTRODUCTION AND ANATOMY

The forearm is made up of 2 bones, the radius and ulna, and has both an anterior and posterior compartment. The muscles of the anterior or flexor compartment of the forearm are largely involved with flexion and pronation. The superficial muscles originate on the common flexor tendon, and the ulnar nerve and artery are also contained within this compartment. The flexor digitorum superficialis lies in between the remaining 4 muscles of the superficial group and the 3 muscles of the deep group; consequently, it is also classified as belonging to the intermediate group. The posterior or extensor compartment of the forearm contains 12 muscles that are chiefly responsible for extension of the wrist and digits and supination of the forearm. The posterior compartment is separated from the anterior compartment by the interosseous membrane that lies between the radius and the ulna.

Most of the muscles that move the wrist, hand, and fingers are located in the forearm. These thin, strap-like muscles extend from the humerus, ulna, and radius, and insert into the carpals, metacarpals, and phalanges via long tendons. The muscles on the anterior side of the forearm, such as the flexor carpi radialis and flexor digitorum superficialis, form the flexor group that flexes the hand at the wrist as well as each of the phalanges.

On the posterior side of the arm, the extensor muscles, such as the extensor carpi ulnaris and extensor digitorum, act as antagonists to the flexor

Grubbs A, ed.
*Taping, Wrapping, and Bracing for Athletic Trainers:
Functional Methods for Application and Fabrication* (pp 135-174).
© 2017 SLACK Incorporated.

muscles by extending the hand and fingers. The extensor muscles run like long, thin straps from the humerus to the metacarpals and phalanges.

The hand and wrist are the most dynamic and complex parts of the upper extremity. There are 8 small carpal bones in the wrist that are firmly bound in 2 rows of 4 bones each. The mass that is made up of these bones is called the carpus. Its distal surface articulates with the metacarpal bones, which are joined to the carpus by the palmar carpometacarpal ligaments.

The 5 long, thin metacarpal bones of the palm extend from the carpus to each of the digits of the hand. The distal heads of the metacarpals are rounded to form condyloid joints with the phalanges (the long, slender bones that form hinge joints between each other) of the fingers. These condyloid joints allow 360-degree motion of the fingers at their bases. Digits 2 to 5 of the hands have 3 phalanges and contain 3 joints each—the proximal interphalangeal joint, interphalangeal joint, and distal interphalangeal joint. The metacarpal has 2 phalanges and contains only 2 joints, the proximal and distal interphalangeal joints.

Common Injuries

Distal Forearm

Wrist Sprain (Hyperextension/Hyperflexion)

An overstretching or tearing of the ligaments of the wrist

Mechanism of Injury

- Falling on an outstretched hand
- Violent, excessive flexion or extension[1] with ulnar or radial deviation
- Abnormal, forced movement of the wrist[1]

Common Signs and Symptoms

- Pain with flexion/extension[1]
- Mild inflammation encapsulating the anterior and posterior aspect of the distal forearm[1]
- Decreased range of motion[1]
- Tenderness over the distal aspect of the forearm

Triangular Fibrocartilaginous Complex Injury

Stretching or tearing of the triangular fibrocartilaginous complex[2]

Mechanism of Injury

- Forced or repeated hyperextension of the wrist
- Compression of the triangular fibrocartilaginous complex[1,2]
- Falling on an outstretched hand[1]

Common Signs and Symptoms

- Pain over the distal to the ulna along the medial half of the wrist[1,2]
- Limited motion into extension[1] and ulnar deviation[2]
- Possible clicking or catching in the wrist upon movement[1,2]
- Possible inflammation[1] over the ulnar aspect of the wrist[2]

Hand

Boxer's Fracture

Fracture to the fifth metacarpal[2]

Mechanism of Injury

- Often a result of a thrown punch

Common Signs and Symptoms

- Depressed fifth metacarpophalangeal joint
- Increased pain
- Decreased range of motion
- Inflammation over the metacarpals of the hand

Scaphoid Fracture

Fracture to the scaphoid that causes instability in the proximal carpal row[2]

Mechanism of Injury

- Forceful hyperextension of the wrist that compresses the scaphoid[2]

Common Signs and Symptoms

- Pain and possible swelling in the anatomical snuffbox[2]
- Pain with radial deviation[2]

- Decreased grip strength[2]
- Decreased strength due to pain[2]

Fingers

Jersey Finger

Avulsion or rupture of the flexor digitorum profundus tendon

Mechanism of Injury

- Violent, traumatic injury caused by a finger getting caught in a uniform
- Axial loaded blunt force trauma

Common Signs and Symptoms

- Point tenderness or pain over the distal interphalangeal joint
- Phalanx remains in extended position
- Inability to actively flex the distal phalanx

Boutonniere Deformity

Avulsion or rupture of the central extensor tendon

Mechanism of Injury

- Longitudinal force on the finger, such as being struck with a ball

Common Signs and Symptoms

- Pain with extension of the distal interphalangeal and metacarpophalangeal joints
- Pain with flexion of the proximal interphalangeal joint
- Pain on the dorsal aspect of the proximal interphalangeal joint

Gamekeeper's/Skier's Thumb

Stretching or tearing of the ulnar collateral ligament of the metacarpophalangeal of the thumb[2]

Mechanism of Injury

- Excessive hyperextension and/or hyperabduction of the first metacarpophalangeal joint[2]

Common Signs and Symptoms

- Pain along the ulnar border of the first metacarpophalangeal joint[2]
- Localized inflammation in the abductor compartment and thenar eminence[2]
- Possible ecchymosis[2]
- Pain with extension, abduction, and opposition[2]
- Decreased range of motion and ability to grip[2]
- Ulnar collateral instability[2]

Phalanx Sprain/Strain

Traumatic overstretching or tearing of the collateral ligaments or tendons of the phalanges[2]

Mechanism of Injury

- Blunt force trauma[2]
- Excessive extension or flexion[2]

Common Signs and Symptoms

- Localized pain at affected joint[2]
- Inflammation[2]
- Decreased range of motion due to pain[2]
- Possible joint deviation

TAPE APPLICATIONS

Forearm

Counterforce Brace

Materials Needed

- Appropriate-sized counterirritant brace

Step 1

Place loosened counterforce brace over the flexor mass of the antebrachial arm (Figure 5-1-1).

Figure 5-1-1.

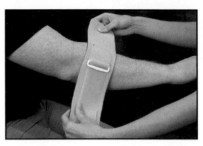

Step 2

Tighten strap with sufficient tension without restricting circulation and without causing neurological dysfunction or pain. Adjust for comfort (Figure 5-1-2).

Figure 5-1-2.

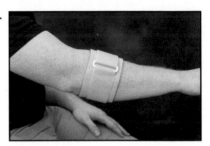

Forearm Sleeve

Materials Needed

- Appropriate-sized compression sleeve/stockinette

Step 1

Place the appropriate-sized forearm sleeve or stockinette over the antebrachial arm (Figure 5-2-1).

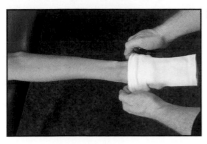

Figure 5-2-1.

Step 2

Once the sleeve is in place, check distal pulse, motor, and sensory function (Figure 5-2-2).

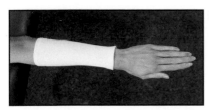

Figure 5-2-2.

Wrist

Tape Jobs

Basic Wrist

Materials Needed

- Adhesive spray (apply prior to taping)
- Prewrap (optional)
- 1.5-inch tape

Step 1

Apply adhesive spray to targeted taping area (Figure 5-3-1).

Figure 5-3-1.

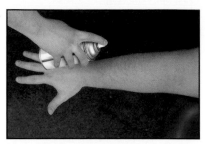

Step 2

Starting 2 to 4 inches proximal to the wrist, apply prewrap, moving distally toward the hand (Figure 5-3-2).

Figure 5-3-2.

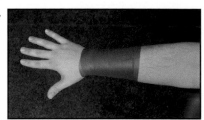

Step 3

Use 1.5-inch white athletic tape and starting 2 to 4 inches proximal to the wrist, place anchor strips. Overlap anchor strips by half the width of the white athletic tape until reaching the distal aspect of the wrist (Figure 5-3-3).

Figure 5-3-3.

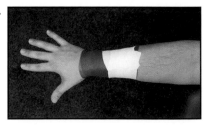

Step 4

Repeat Step 2 until desired limit in range of motion restriction is achieved (Figure 5-3-4).

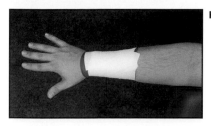

Figure 5-3-4.

Step 5

Check for capillary refill (Figure 5-3-5).

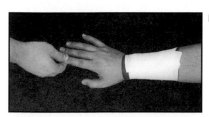

Figure 5-3-5.

Please refer to the Basic Wrist tape job (Video) for further review and variation preference in performing this taping technique.

Wrist Through Hand

Materials Needed

- Adhesive spray (apply prior to taping)
- Prewrap (optional)
- 1.5-inch tape

Step 1

Apply adhesive spray to targeted taping area (Figure 5-4-1).

Figure 5-4-1.

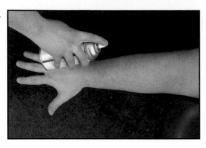

Step 2

Starting 2 to 4 inches proximal to the wrist, apply prewrap, moving distally toward the hand (Figure 5-4-2).

Figure 5-4-2.

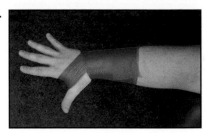

Step 3

Using 1.5-inch white athletic tape and starting 2 to 4 inches proximal to the wrist, place anchor strips. Overlap anchor strips by half the width of the white athletic tape until reaching the distal aspect of the wrist (Figure 5-4-3).

Figure 5-4-3.

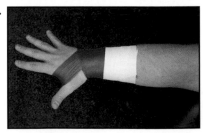

Step 4

Beginning at the dorsal aspect of the wrist, angle the tape toward the thenar eminence of the hand, moving toward the palmar aspect, until reaching the wrist anchor strips (Figure 5-4-4).

Note: Be sure to slightly pinch the tape as it passes over the thenar eminence to prevent irritation.

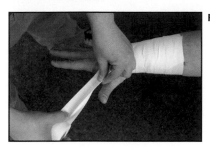

Figure 5-4-4.

Step 5

Repeat Step 2, either 2 or 3 more times, and secure to the wrist with anchor strips (Figure 5-4-5).

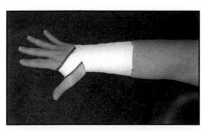

Figure 5-4-5.

Step 6

Continue with anchor strips around the wrist until desired support is achieved (Figure 5-4-6).

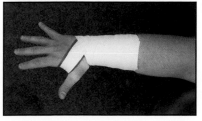

Figure 5-4-6.

Step 7

Check for range of motion and capillary refill (Figure 5-4-7).

Figure 5-4-7.

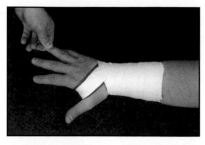

Please refer to the Through the Hand tape job (Video) for further review and variation preference in performing this taping technique.

Wrist Diamond

Materials Needed

- Adhesive spray (optional)
- Prewrap
- 1.5-inch white athletic tape

Step 1

Starting 2 to 4 inches proximal to the wrist, apply adhesive spray and prewrap, moving distally toward the hand (Figure 5-5-1).

Figure 5-5-1.

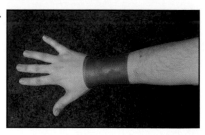

Step 2

Using 1.5-inch white athletic tape and starting 2 to 4 inches proximal to the wrist, move distally until the wrist is sufficiently covered (Figure 5-5-2).

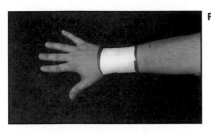

Figure 5-5-2.

Step 3

Starting at the posterior aspect of the wrist, angle the tape proximally, wrapping around the wrist and returning to the starting point on the wrist (Figure 5-5-3).

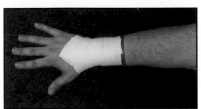

Figure 5-5-3.

Step 4

Repeat Step 2 until desired limit in range of motion restriction is achieved.

Note: Angled strips will give the final product a diamond pattern.

Step 5

Secure the diamond with anchor strips over the wrist, closing the tape job (Figure 5-5-4).

Figure 5-5-4.

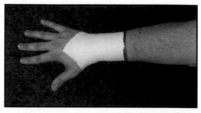

Step 6

Check for capillary refill (Figure 5-5-5).

Figure 5-5-5.

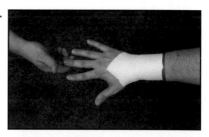

Please refer to the Wrist Diamond tape job (Video) for further review and variation preference in performing this taping technique.

Wrist Hyperextension

Materials Needed

- Adhesive spray (apply prior to taping)
- Prewrap (optional)
- Scissors
- 1.5-inch white athletic tape

Step 1

Starting 2 to 4 inches proximal to the wrist, apply prewrap, moving distally toward the hand (Figure 5-6-1).

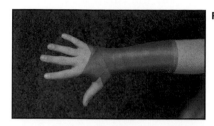

Figure 5-6-1.

Step 2

Using 1.5-inch white athletic tape and starting 2 to 4 inches proximal to the wrist, move distally until the wrist is sufficiently covered. Be sure to overlap by half the width of the tape as you move distally (Figure 5-6-2).

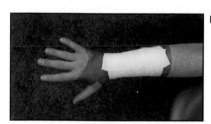

Figure 5-6-2.

Step 3

Place an anchor strip through the hand. If necessary, pinch the tape to prevent irritation of the webbing of the thenar space (Figure 5-6-3).

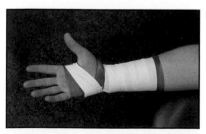

Figure 5-6-3.

Step 4

Create an X shape with 2 strips of the 1.5-inch tape and then add the third strip vertically on top of the X (this will be referred to as a fan). Using the scissors, round off the ends of the fan. This will ensure a cleaner tape job (Figure 5-6-4).

Figure 5-6-4.

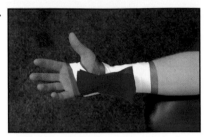

Step 5

On the palmar aspect of the wrist, apply the fan to the anchor strip around the hand and secure with cover strips (Figure 5-6-5).

Figure 5-6-5.

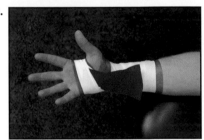

Step 6

Pulling proximally, attach the fan on the anchor strips of the wrist (Figure 5-6-6).

Figure 5-6-6.

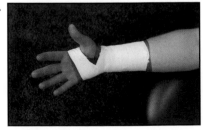

Step 7

Secure the fan with an anchor over the wrist and close the tape job (Figure 5-6-7).

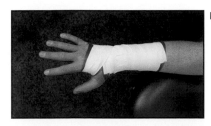

Figure 5-6-7.

Step 8

Check for proper range of motion and capillary refill (Figure 5-6-8).

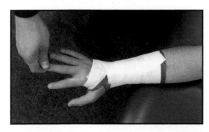

Figure 5-6-8.

Please refer to the Wrist Hyperextension tape job (Video) for further review and variation preference in performing this taping technique.

Wrist Hyperflexion

Materials Needed

- Adhesive spray (apply prior to taping)
- Prewrap (optional)
- Scissors
- 1.5-inch white athletic tape

Step 1

Apply adhesive spray to targeted taping area. Starting 2 to 4 inches proximal to the wrist, apply prewrap, moving distally toward the hand (Figure 5-7-1).

Figure 5-7-1.

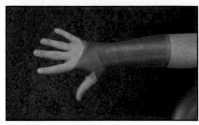

Step 2

Using 1.5-inch white athletic tape, and starting 2 to 4 inches proximal to the wrist, move distally until the wrist is sufficiently covered. Be sure to overlap by half the width of the tape as you move distally (Figure 5-7-2).

Figure 5-7-2.

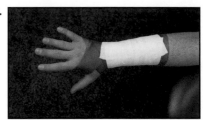

Step 3

Place an anchor strip through the hand. If necessary, pinch the tape to prevent irritation of the webbing of the thenar space (Figure 5-7-3).

Figure 5-7-3.

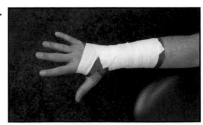

Step 4

Create an X shape with 2 strips of the 1.5-inch tape and then add the third strip of tape vertically on top of the X (this is referred to as a fan). Using the scissors, round off the ends of the fan. This will ensure a cleaner tape job (Figure 5-7-4).

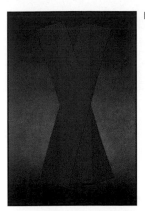

Figure 5-7-4.

Step 5

On the dorsal aspect of the hand, apply the fan to the distal aspect of the wrist and secure with an anchor strip (Figure 5-7-5).

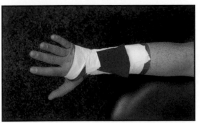

Figure 5-7-5.

Step 6

Pulling proximally, attach the fan on the anchor strips of the wrist (Figure 5-7-6).

Figure 5-7-6.

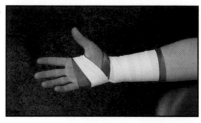

Step 7

Secure the fan with an anchor over the wrist and close the tape job (Figure 5-7-7).

Figure 5-7-7.

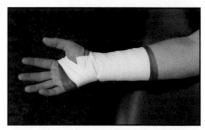

Step 8

Have the athlete flex and extend the wrist to check for desired range of motion (Figure 5-7-8).

Figure 5-7-8.

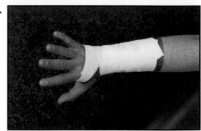

Check for capillary refill (Figure 5-7-9).

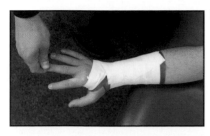

Figure 5-7-9.

Please refer to the Wrist Hyperflexion tape job (Video) for further review and variation preference in performing this taping technique.

Braces

Wrist Brace With Thumb

Materials Needed

- Appropriate-sized wrist brace with thumb support
- Prewrap
- 1.5-inch white athletic tape
- 2-inch stretch tape

Step 1

Place the brace on the wrist, making sure the straps are loose (Figure 5-8-1).

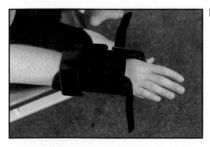

Figure 5-8-1.

Step 2

Once properly adjusted on the wrist, fasten straps to ensure a snug fit. Follow the adjustment by applying prewrap over the fitted brace (Figure 5-8-2).

Figure 5-8-2.

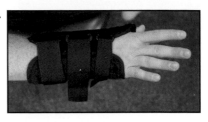

Step 3

Cover the brace with 2-inch stretch tape to keep straps fastened, covering the thumb portion if needed. Use 1.5-inch white athletic tape to anchor and complete the tape job (Figure 5-8-3).

Figure 5-8-3.

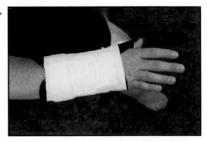

Step 4

Check for capillary refill (Figure 5-8-4).

Figure 5-8-4.

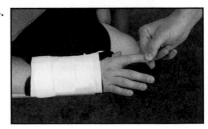

Fingers

Thumb Spica

Materials Needed

- Adhesive spray (apply prior to taping)
- Prewrap (optional)
- 1-inch white athlete tape
- 1.5-inch white athletic tape

Step 1

Shake the athlete's hand to put it in the proper position.

Step 2

Apply adhesive spray to targeted taping area. Starting 2 to 4 inches proximal to the wrist, apply prewrap, moving through the hand and around the thumb (Figure 5-9-1).

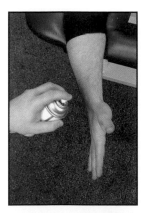

Figure 5-9-1.

Step 3

Using 1.5-inch white athletic tape, place 2 anchor strips around the distal wrist (Figure 5-9-2).

Figure 5-9-2.

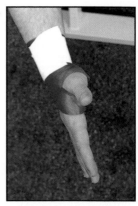

Step 4

Beginning at the posterior aspect of the wrist, cross the 1-inch white athletic tape over the metacarpophalangeal joint, around the thumb, and back across the metacarpophalangeal joint, finishing on the anterior aspect of the wrist (Figure 5-9-3).

Figure 5-9-3.

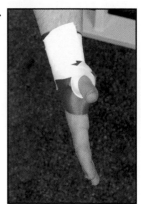

Step 5

Beginning at the anterior aspect of the wrist, cross the 1-inch white athletic tape over the metacarpophalangeal joint, around the thumb, and back across the metacarpophalangeal joint, finishing on the posterior aspect of the wrist (Figure 5-9-4).

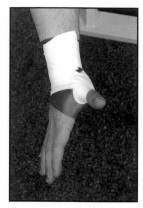

Figure 5-9-4.

Step 6

Repeat Steps 4 and 5, either 2 or 3 times, overlapping the tape by half the width each time or until the thumb is covered to the distal phalangeal joint (Figure 5-9-5).

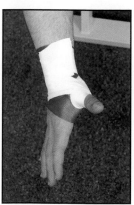

Figure 5-9-5.

Step 7

Close the tape job with 1.5-inch anchor strips to secure the spica (Figure 5-9-6).

Note: Be sure to slightly pinch the tape as it passes over the webbing between the thumb and index finger to prevent irritation.

Figure 5-9-6.

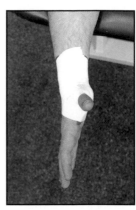

Step 8

Check for capillary refill (Figure 5-9-7).

Figure 5-9-7.

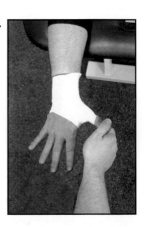

Please refer to the Thumb Spica tape job (Video) for further review and variation preference in performing this taping technique.

Modified Thumb Spica

Materials Needed

- Adhesive (apply prior to taping)
- Prewrap (optional)
- 1-inch white athletic tape
- 1.5-inch white athletic tape

Step 1

Apply adhesive spray and prewrap to targeted area (Figure 5-10-1).

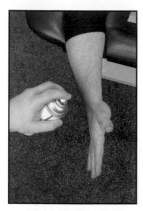

Figure 5-10-1.

Step 2

Using 1.5-inch white athletic tape, place 2 to 3 anchor strips around the distal wrist (Figure 5-10-2).

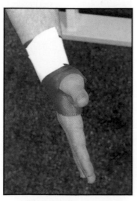

Figure 5-10-2.

Step 3

Beginning at the posterior aspect of the wrist, cross the 1-inch white athletic tape over the metacarpophalangeal joint, around the thumb, and back across the metacarpophalangeal joint, finishing on the posterior aspect of the wrist (Figure 5-10-3).

Figure 5-10-3.

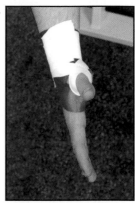

Step 4

Repeat Step 3, either 3 or 4 times, overlapping the tape by half the width each time or until the thumb is covered to the middle phalangeal joint (Figure 5-10-4).

Figure 5-10-4.

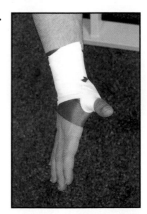

Step 5

Using 1.5-inch white athletic tape, place 2 to 3 C strips at the base of the first metacarpal and move distally (Figure 5-10-5).

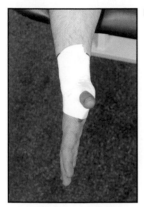

Figure 5-10-5.

Step 6

Using 1.5-inch white athletic tape, place a C strip through the thenar eminence (shown in red; Figure 5-10-6).

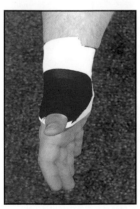

Figure 5-10-6.

Step 7

Close the tape job with anchor strips to secure the spica (Figure 5-10-7).

Figure 5-10-7.

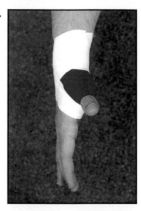

Step 8

Check for capillary refill (Figure 5-10-8).

Figure 5-10-8.

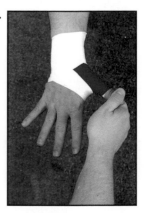

Please refer to the Thumb Alternative and Modified Thumb Spica tape jobs (Videos) for further review and variation preference in performing these taping techniques.

Buddy Tape

Materials Needed

- Adhesive spray (apply prior to taping)
- 0.5-inch tape

Step 1

Align the injured finger next to the adjacent healthy finger (Figure 5-11-1).

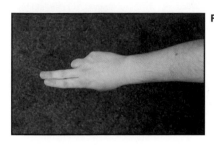

Figure 5-11-1.

Step 2

Using 0.5-inch white athletic tape, make an anchor between the metacarpophalangeal and proximal interphalangeal joints (Figure 5-11-2).

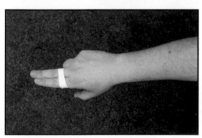

Figure 5-11-2.

Step 3

Place another 0.5-inch white athletic tape anchor strip between the proximal interphalangeal and distal interphalangeal joints (Figure 5-11-3).

Figure 5-11-3.

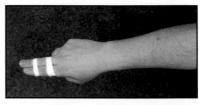

Step 4

If necessary, repeat Steps 2 and 3 until adequate support has been achieved.

Step 5

Check for capillary refill (Figure 5-11-4).

Figure 5-11-4.

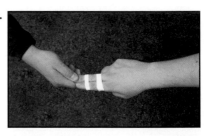

Please refer to the Buddy Tape tape job (Video) for further review and variation preference in performing this taping technique.

Boxer Tape

Materials Needed

- Adhesive spray (apply prior to taping)
- Prewrap (optional)
- 0.5-inch white athletic tape
- 1-inch rolled gauze
- 1.5-inch white athletic tape
- 2-inch stretch tape

Step 1

Apply adhesive spray and prewrap to targeted area (Figure 5-12-1).

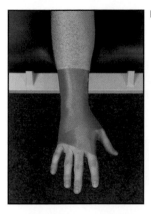

Figure 5-12-1.

Step 2

Using 1.5-inch white athletic tape and starting 2 to 4 inches proximal to the wrist, place anchor strips. Overlap anchor strips by half the width of the white athletic tape until reaching the distal aspect of the wrist. Beginning at the palmar aspect of the wrist, angle the tape toward the thenar eminence of the hand, moving dorsally until reaching the wrist anchor strips (Figure 5-12-2).

Note: Be sure to slightly pinch the tape as it passes over the thenar eminence to prevent irritation.

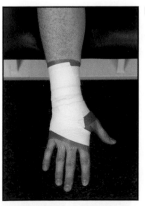

Figure 5-12-2.

Step 3

Next, using 1-inch gauze and starting at the palmar aspect of the wrist, angle toward the thenar eminence of the hand. Come back through the medial aspect of the fourth phalanx. Pass over the palmar aspect of the wrist with the gauze and angle toward the lateral aspect of the third phalanx, wrapping around the palmar aspect of the wrist and coming back up around the medial aspect of the third phalanx. Pass over the palmar aspect of the wrist with the gauze and angle toward the lateral aspect of the second phalanx, wrapping around the palmar aspect of the wrist and coming back up around the medial aspect of the second phalanx (Figure 5-12-3).

Figure 5-12-3.

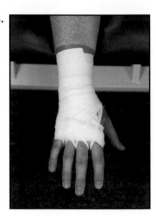

Step 4

Following the application of the gauze, utilize 0.5-inch tape to create anchors between each webspace of the phalanges (Figure 5-12-4).

Figure 5-12-4.

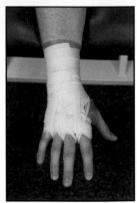

Step 5

Use 2-inch stretch tape to close the tape job (Figure 5-12-5).

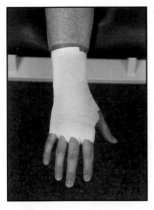

Figure 5-12-5.

Step 6

Check for capillary refill (Figure 5-12-6).

Note: This tape job is not strictly pertained for boxers but can be utilized for athletes who are primarily physical with their hands. This is strictly a variation of an actual boxer's tape job.

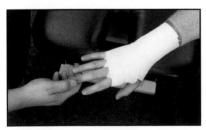

Figure 5-12-6.

Please refer to the Boxer tape job (Video) for further review and variation preference in performing this taping technique.

Single Finger Tape

Materials Needed

- Adhesive spray (apply prior to taping)
- 0.5-inch white athletic tape

Step 1

Spray adhesive spray to targeted taping area. Allow to dry and become tacky (Figure 5-13-1).

Figure 5-13-1.

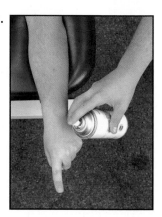

Step 2

Start with an anchor strip in-between the metacarpal and proximal interphalangeal joints.

Then place another anchor strip between the proximal interphalangeal and distal interphalangeal joints (Figure 5-13-2).

Figure 5-13-2.

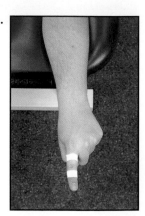

Step 3

Start the tape on the anterior aspect of the proximal anchor; laying it medially, cross over the proximal interphalangeal joint and attach the end to the posterior aspect of the distal anchor (Figure 5-13-3).

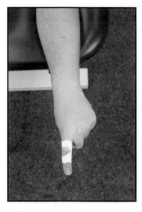

Figure 5-13-3.

Step 4

Next, start the tape on the posterior aspect of the proximal anchor; laying it medially, cross over the proximal interphalangeal joint, and attach the end to the anterior aspect of the distal anchor (Figure 5-13-4).

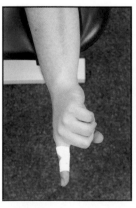

Figure 5-13-4.

Step 5

Again, start the tape on the anterior aspect of the proximal anchor; laying it laterally, cross over the proximal interphalangeal joint and attach the end to the posterior aspect of the distal anchor (Figure 5-13-5).

Figure 5-13-5.

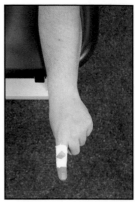

Step 6

Next, start the tape on the posterior aspect of the proximal anchor; laying it laterally, cross over the proximal interphalangeal joint and attach the end to the anterior aspect of the distal anchor (Figure 5-13-6).

Figure 5-13-6.

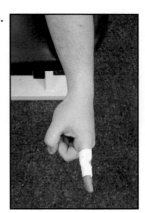

Step 7

Repeat Steps 4 through 7, making an X pattern over the collateral ligaments of the finger until the desired level of support is achieved.

Step 8

Lastly, place another anchor strip over both the proximal and distal anchors to secure the collateral support X's (Figure 5-13-7).

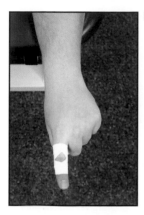

Figure 5-13-7.

Step 9

Check for capillary refill (Figure 5-13-8).

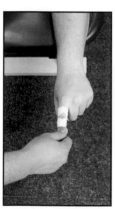

Figure 5-13-8.

Please refer to the Finger Tape tape job (Video) for further review and variation preference in performing this taping technique.

REFERENCES

1. Prentice WE. *Arnheim's Principles of Athletic Training: A Competency-Based Approach.* 14th ed. New York, NY: McGraw-Hill; 2010.
2. Starkey C, Brown SD. *Examination of Orthopedic and Athletic Injuries.* 4th ed. Philadelphia, PA: FA Davis Co; 2015.

Please see videos on the accompanying website at
www.healio.com/books/tapingAT

6

Orthoplast

COMMON INJURIES

Orthoplast (Johnson & Johnson) has been used to create a pliable padding cover that can move with the joints and body parts through the necessary range of motion, but still protect the affected area of the body in static positions. Orthoplast offers the following advantages: it is lightweight, provides rigid protection, and is form fitting.[1] This form-fitting nature makes Orthoplast an aerodynamic product ideal for athletes in speed sports. It offers more padding than foam or felt, making it much more suited to high-velocity, high-impact sports.[1] In medical settings, this material can be used in a variety of ways, such as for temporary braces, corrective bracing devices, and supportive braces. Doctors and allied health professionals use Orthoplast to make custom-fitted braces that provide comfort and support without injuring the body.

This product is an example of a thermoplastic. A thermoplastic is a type of plastic made from polymer resins that becomes a homogenized liquid when heated and hard when cooled. These characteristics lend the material its name and make it recyclable. Moreover, the effects are reversible—in other words, thermoplastics can be reheated, reshaped, and frozen repeatedly. When heated, Orthoplast is malleable, with an almost rubbery texture, and can be molded around the area of the body being braced or splinted. As it cools, the material hardens, creating a brace that fits perfectly.

Grubbs A, ed.
*Taping, Wrapping, and Bracing for Athletic Trainers:
Functional Methods for Application and Fabrication* (pp 175-187).
© 2017 SLACK Incorporated.

Orthoplast comes in perforated varieties (to allow air circulation) as well as plain sheets and is usually white. It is generally recommended that padding be used under a brace to distribute pressure, prevent sores, and increase patient comfort. Additionally, Orthoplast must be filed once it is fitted so that any sharp edges do not gouge the patient. It can be attached to tapes, rods, rivets, and other devices used to fix it in place.

One advantage to Orthoplast is that it can be used to make a custom brace of any size. It can also be used for other purposes, such as creating custom lightweight splints for injured fingers.

An orthopedic surgeon may utilize Orthoplast as part of a cast or for bracing when a body part has been removed from a cast, but still requires support. It can also be used to manage stress and strain on a limb and for corrective bracing designed to address issues such as poor posture or abnormal growth patterns. It is important that a trained health care professional—one who can confirm that the fit is correct and so minimize the risk of injury to the patient—supervise the fitting of Orthoplast. Since only high temperatures will mold Orthoplast, the proper equipment, such as a hydrocollator, is needed to heat it.

Orthoplast Uses

Shoulder

Acromioclavicular Pad

Materials Needed

- Orthoplast
- Scissors
- Soft foam padding
- Hydrocollator

Step 1

Cut a square out of the Orthoplast fit to the size of the athlete's shoulder and begin to heat.

Tip: Use a sheet of paper to get the proper shape size before cutting the Orthoplast.

Step 2

Use an item such as half a golf ball or the cardboard center of a tape roll to create a dome-like indention into the Orthoplast above the acromioclavicular joint (Figure 6-1-1).

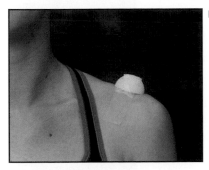

Figure 6-1-1.

Step 3

Once the Orthoplast is pliable, mold and shape it to the curvature of the athlete's shoulder (Figure 6-1-2).

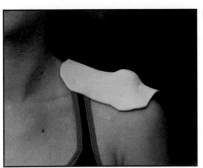

Figure 6-1-2.

Step 4

Once the Orthoplast hardens, mark the directions in order to line it back up later (Figure 6-1-3).

Figure 6-1-3.

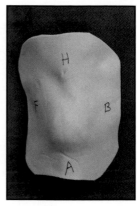

Step 5

Add a soft foam padding layer to the underside to prevent irritation and to provide additional comfort to the athlete (Figure 6-1-4).

Figure 6-1-4.

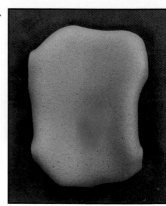

Step 6

Smooth down the edges, heating only these areas to help prevent irritation (Figure 6-1-5).

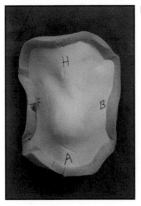

Figure 6-1-5.

Step 7

Use the shoulder spica wrap for securing (Figure 6-1-6).

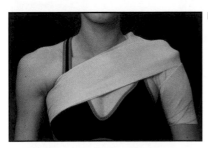

Figure 6-1-6.

Wrist Hyperextension

Wrist

Materials Needed

- Moleskin
- Orthoplast
- Scissors
- Soft foam padding
- Hydrocollator

Step 1

Cut a rectangle out of the Orthoplast to the size of the patient's wrist, and begin to heat. Size may need to be adjusted based on the size of the athlete's wrist (Figure 6-2-1).

Tip: Use a sheet of paper to get the proper shape size before cutting the Orthoplast.

Figure 6-2-1.

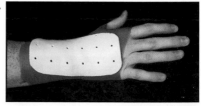

Step 2

Once the Orthoplast is pliable, mold and shape it to fit the curvature of the athlete's wrist (Figure 6-2-2).

Figure 6-2-2.

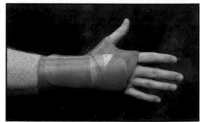

Step 3

Once the Orthoplast hardens, add a soft foam padding layer to the underside to prevent irritation and to provide additional comfort to the athlete.

Step 4

Smooth down the edges, heating only these areas to help prevent irritation (Figure 6-2-3).

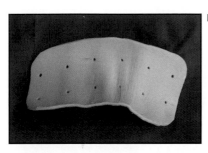

Figure 6-2-3.

Step 5

Lastly, moleskin can be used around the edges of the wrist pad to protect the athlete from irritation (Figures 6-2-4A and B).

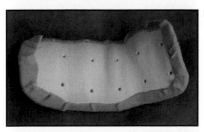

Figure 6-2-4A.

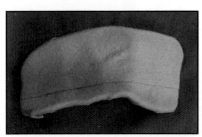

Figure 6-2-4B.

Thumb Spica

Materials Needed

- Moleskin
- Orthoplast
- Prewrap
- Scissors
- Hydrocollator

Step 1

Cut a teardrop out of the Orthoplast to a size that will cover the patient's thumb. Then begin to heat the Orthoplast (Figure 6-3-1).

Tip: Use a sheet of paper to get the proper shape size before cutting the Orthoplast.

Figure 6-3-1.

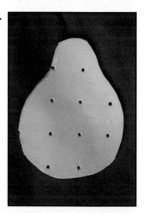

Step 2

Cover the patient's hand, wrist, and thumb in prewrap (Figure 6-3-2).

Figure 6-3-2.

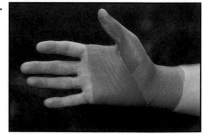

Step 3

Once the Orthoplast is pliable, mold and shape it around the thumb, ensuring that it extends past the proximal interphalangeal joint (Figure 6-3-3).

Note: If elected to mold Orthoplast past the wrist joint, ensure the wrist is in the desired position before the splint hardens.

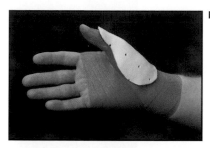

Figure 6-3-3.

Step 4

By heating only these areas, smooth down the edges to help prevent irritation (Figure 6-3-4).

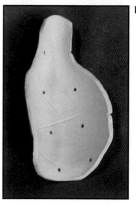

Figure 6-3-4.

Step 5

Lastly, moleskin can be used around the thumb spica splint to protect the athlete from irritation (Figures 6-3-5A and B).

Figure 6-3-5A.

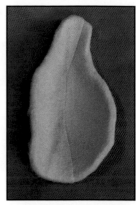

Figure 6-3-5B.

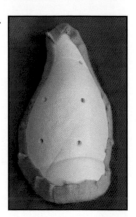

Step 6

Prewrap the athlete's thumb to provide a thin layer of padding and reduce friction (Figure 6-3-6).

Refer to thumb spica taping techniques for application of the Orthoplast once it has been molded to the thumb.

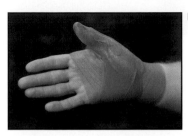

Figure 6-3-6.

Please refer to the Thumb Spica tape job (Video) for further review and variation preference in performing this taping technique.

Soft Cast Thumb/Wrist

Materials Needed

- Gloves
- Moleskin
- 2-inch soft cast
- Prewrap
- Scissors
- Tepid water
- Lotion (optional)

Note: For application of the soft cast, make sure to wear gloves.

Step 1

Starting 2 to 4 inches proximal to the wrist, apply prewrap, moving through the hand and around the thumb (Figure 6-4-1).

Figure 6-4-1.

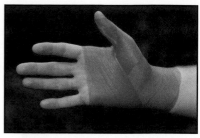

Step 2

Dampen the soft cast material with tepid water, and apply from the proximal to distal end of the wrist, going through the hand and around the thumb. Make sure to smooth down the cast once it is applied so that there are no rough edges that could potentially harm the athlete. Water or lotion can be utilized to smooth down the cast (Figure 6-4-2).

Figure 6-4-2.

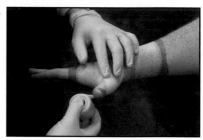

Step 3

The hand should be covered from the metacarpophalangeal joint to the wrist and the thumb covered to the distal interphalangeal joint (Figure 6-4-3).

Figure 6-4-3.

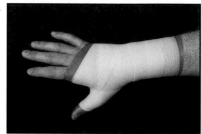

Step 4

A cut should be made across the medial side of the soft cast (along the little finger side of the cast) so that it can be utilized during future games and events (Figure 6-4-4).

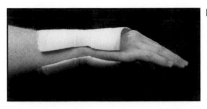

Figure 6-4-4.

Step 5

Moleskin can be used around the inside of the soft cast to protect the athlete from irritation.

REFERENCE

1.   Snouse SL, Lundgren KL. Use of Orthoplast for winter sports. *J Athl Train.* 1998;28(3):230-235.

Glossary

ANATOMICAL POSITIONING

- Anterior: toward the front (Figure G-1)
- Posterior: toward the back (Figure G-1)

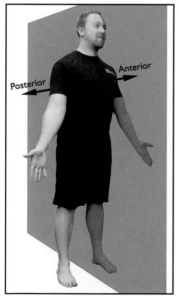

Figure G-1.

Grubbs A, ed.
*Taping, Wrapping, and Bracing for Athletic Trainers:
Functional Methods for Application and Fabrication* (pp 189-195).
© 2017 SLACK Incorporated.

- Superior: closer to the head (Figure G-2)
- Inferior: closer to the toes (Figure G-2)

Figure G-2.

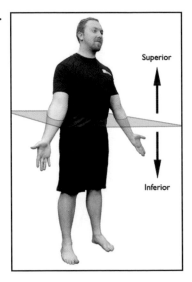

- Deep: a part that is more internal (Figure G-3)
- Superficial: toward the surface (Figure G-3)

Figure G-3.

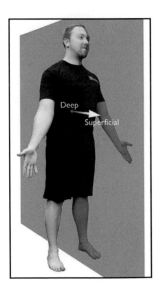

- Medial: toward the midline of the body (imaginary line that divides the body into equal halves; Figure G-4)
- Lateral: away from the midline of the body (Figure G-4)

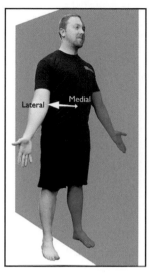

Figure G-4.

- Ipsilateral: the same side
- Contralateral: the opposite side
- Proximal: closer to the trunk (Figure G-5)
- Distal: far from the trunk (Figure G-5)

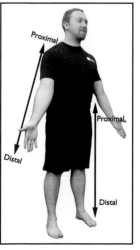

Figure G-5.

- Abduction: away from the body (Figure G-6)
- Adduction: toward the body (Figure G-6)

Figure G-6.

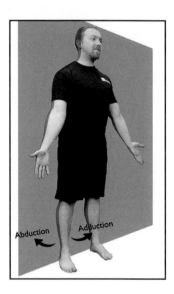

- Horizontal adduction: decreasing the angle across the body along the transverse plane
- Horizontal abduction: increasing the angle across the body along the transverse plane
- Inversion: turning inward when pertaining to the foot
- Eversion: turning outward when pertaining to the foot
- Flexion: decreasing the angle of the joint
- Extension: increasing the angle of the joint
- Dorsiflexion: flexion of the foot in an upward direction
- Plantar flexion: flexion of the foot in a downward direction

- Planes of the body (Figure G-7)

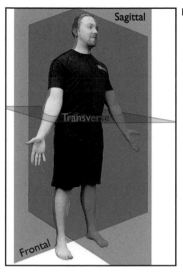

Figure G-7.

- Transverse/horizontal plane: divides the body into superior and inferior portions (Figure G-8)

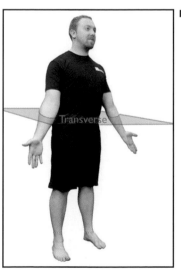

Figure G-8.

- Sagittal plane: divides the body into equal left and right halves (Figure G-9)

Figure G-9.

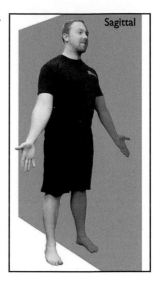

- Frontal plane: divides the body into anterior and posterior portions (Figure G-10)

Figure G-10.

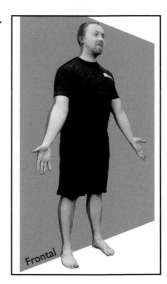

Miscellaneous

- Gait: manner of walking, running, or jogging
- Triceps surae: gastrocnemius and the soleus
- Neuroma: a tumor or mass growing from a nerve and usually consisting of nerve fibers
- Strain: tear in a muscle or tendon
- Sprain: tear in a ligament
- Antalgic gait: abnormal manner of walking, running, or jogging
- Q-angle: determines the approximate tracking of the patella through the relationship between the anterior superior iliac spine, the midpoint, and the tibial tuberosity; helps quantify the line of pull of the quad on the patellar tendon, resulting in force on the patella[1]

Reference

1. Starkey C, Brown SD. *Examination of Orthopedic and Athletic Injuries.* 4th ed. Philadelphia, PA: FA Davis Co; 2015.

Financial Disclosures

The editor, associate editors, and contributing authors of *Taping, Wrapping, and Bracing for Athletic Trainers: Functional Methods for Application and Fabrication* would like to acknowledge and thank the following listed companies who provided tape and braces for this project. Other than this in-kind support, the editor, associate editors, and contributing authors have no relevant financial relationships to report with these companies listed below:

- Bledsoe
- Breg
- DonJoy
- Medco
- United Sports Brands

Index